Dr. Sebi Recipe Book:

101 Tasty and Easy-Made Cell Foods for Detox, Cleanse, and Revitalizing Your Body and Soule Using the Dr. Sebi Food List and Products

Table of Contents

Introduction

I would like to thank you for choosing *Dr. Sebi Recipe Book*. This book will provide you with 101 delicious recipes that you can enjoy as you follow Dr. Sebi's diet.

For those of you who do not know, Dr. Sebi was a naturalist, biochemist, herbalist, and pathologist. During his life, he studied herbs throughout the Caribbean, Africa, and all of America. Through his studies, he came up with his own methodology and approach to healing the body with herbs.

He was born on November 26, 1933, as Alfredo Bowman in Ilanga Village in Honduras. He was completely self-educated and learned a lot from his grandmother. During his childhood, he would play in the forest and by the river and learned a lot about nature.

After he made his move to the United States, he was diagnosed with obesity, impotency, diabetes, and asthma, but modern medicine couldn't help him. This led him to travel to Mexico to see an herbalist. He found great success with this route, and he started to create natural methods of healing the cells in the body. He dedicated more than 30 years of his life coming up with his own methodology. This is how he gave birth to Dr. Sebi's Cell Food.

His teachings have disputed germ theory. Dr. Sebi did not believe that our ailments were caused by germs, bacteria, viruses, and so on. He believed that the root of all of our problems was an excess of mucus in the system. Many of his teachings were Afrocentric and focused on the unique genetic characteristics of Africans.

Dr. Sebi had a practice in New York and then opened USHA Research Institute in Usha Village in Honduras. Throughout his years, he has worked with lots of celebrities. Wendy

Williams once took her son, Kevin Jr., to Usha Village to help him after he used synthetic marijuana.

TLCs Lisa Lopes also visited Usha Village during her short time. This was also where she had been when she was in her unfortunate accident. He also helped treat Michael Jackson, Nipsey Hussle, John Travolta, Steven Seagal, and Eddie Murphy.

In 1988, Dr. Sebi was faced with a Supreme Court trial for false advertisement and practicing without a license. This happened after he had placed ads in several newspapers. The judge asked Dr. Sebi to produce one person for each disease. He said that he could cure. When the trial started, Dr. Sebi brought in 77 people. The juror ended up ruling in his favor and found him not guilty. After this, he moved his practice to LA.

He continued to thrive even after the lawsuit. Unfortunately, he was faced with another lawsuit. He was arrested on May 28, 2016, in Honduras for money laundering. He was never able to defend himself in this matter because he died of complications with pneumonia at the age of 82 while in police custody.

Despite these setbacks, Dr. Sebi still lives on in the hearts of those he has helped and continues to help.

Disclaimer

Please note that we are not doctors and we do not claim to be. We simply follow the instructions of Dr. Sebi.

Chapter 1: Eating Naturally with Dr. Sebi's Teachings

The Dr. Sebi diet is often referred to as the African biomineral balance. This was how he would cure people of a variety of diseases. It is basically a vegan diet that is made up of foods that he called "electric" or alkaline foods. It is suggested that, while following this diet, you also take his healing supplements.

You cannot eat any meat or animal products while on this diet, as well as foods that contain a lot of starch. The reason for this is that you are only supposed to eat alkaline-forming foods, and those foods form acids.

Meat products cause uric acid production, dairy produces cause lactic acid, and starch causes carbonic acid. All of these acids will build-up, which causes a buildup of mucus. The mucus robs our cells of oxygen. However, if you eat electric foods, they feed the body. The human body is electrical, so it needs electric food to function.

This diet is made up of grains, teas, nuts, veggies, and fruits. Among the foods you can eat are wild rice, amaranth, quinoa, mushrooms, watercress, kale, dates, figs, mangos, avocados, and much more. These foods will help to nourish your body and won't end up causing an accumulation of mucus.

If you plan on really starting this diet, you must make sure that you really want it. The first thing you will need to do is to make some changes to how you eat. You will probably find that this is going to require you to be your best emotional state and the right state of mind.

Eating is a big part of our life, and the types of things we consume form strong habits that can end up lasting our entire life. It can be very hard to break these habits and deal with the influence of family and friends. That means, before you jump right into this diet, you should take some time thinking about changing how you eat. You don't want to promise yourself this and then end up not being able to follow through just because you weren't prepared.

Instead, you should begin slowly. You can even talk to your family and friends. The reaction you can get from people when you talk to them about Dr. Sebi's diet will vary. Some will want to learn more, while others will write it off as bunk.

That being said, you shouldn't tire yourself by trying to convince everybody else before you make sure that it is right for you. Your vitality, health improvements, and cleaner outlook will show your family way more than just your words.

Once you do start making the transition, the first thing you need to do is to start reading food ingredient labels on everything. This will help you to stay conscious about what you are drinking and eating. When you are first starting out, before you live completely by the nutritional guide, this awareness is going to provide you with the incentive to change things as you continue on. Later on, if you do end up straying from the diet, you will still be able to remain conscious about what you are eating.

If you have long been a meat-eater, that may be the hardest thing to transition from. The best thing you can do is to start making the transition from meats by switching to eating only fish. Then you can slowly start eating less and less fish each week.

It is also important that you start making your own snacks. This will ensure if you do get the urge to snack, that you will have good snacks to eat. Approved nuts and raisins are a good choice.

Then you need to make sure that you are eating all of the correct foods. That means you need to learn what foods are and aren't on the nutritional guide. You must stick to only those foods. At first, this will feel tough, and that is expected. In fact, it is very hard to do in our society when only the bad foods are pushed at us. This is the reason why I stressed that you must be emotionally ready.

You also need to make sure you are drinking plenty of water. While we have all known for a while now that water is a very important part of our health, most of us are still not drink enough. Plus, there are a lot of Dr. Sebi products that you will be taking, like the Bromide Plus Powder, contain herbs that act as diuretics. That means you have to take extra care to make sure you don't allow yourself to get dehydrated.

Dr. Sebi suggests that you drink a gallon of spring water every day. Springwater has a natural alkaline pH, whereas tap water can be high in chloride and many other contaminants.

You will also need to learn how to cook your own meals if you don't cook already. You aren't going to find too many prepackaged foods that fit into the Dr. Sebi diet. Once you do get the hang of cooking, you will find that you can change your favorite dishes into Dr. Sebi-approved dishes.

Chapter 2: Alkaline Meals

Salads and Soups

Basil and Cucumber Gazpacho

What you'll need:

- Key lime juice, 1 lime

- Sea salt, 1.25 tsp.

- Water, 2 c

- Fresh basil, 2 handfuls

- Cucumber, 1 seeded

- Avocado, 1

What you'll do:

Put all the ingredients into the refrigerator and leave until chilled.

Once everything is cold, put them into the blender and turn on until creamy and smooth.

Put the soup back into the refrigerator until you are ready to serve.

When you are ready to eat, ladle into bowls and garnish with basil leaves and cucumber slices.

Citrus Watercress Salad

What you'll need:

- Cayenne pepper, to taste
- Salt, dash
- Olive oil, 2 tbsp
- Juice of one key lime
- Agave syrup, 2 tsp.
- Thinly sliced red onion, 2
- Zest of one Seville orange
- Segments of Seville orange
- Watercress, 4 c
- Avocado, 1

What you'll do:

Take two plates and divide out the orange segments, sliced onions, sliced avocados, and watercress evenly.

In a small bowl, place the cayenne pepper, salt, agave syrup, olive oil, and lime juice. Whisk until well combined.

Pour over salad once you are ready to serve.

Sloppy Joe

What you'll need:

- Grapeseed oil
- Cayenne pepper, pinch
- Sea salt, 1 tsp.
- Diced plum tomato
- Onion powder, 1 tsp.
- Diced green bell peppers, .5 c
- Diced onion, .5 c
- Cooked garbanzo beans, 1 c
- Barbecue sauce, 1.5 c
- Cooked Kamut or spelt, 2 c
- Barbecue Sauce:
- Cloves, pinch
- Onion powder, 2 tsp.
- Cayenne, .25 tsp.
- Ground ginger, .5 tsp.
- Sea salt, 2 tsp.
- Chopped white onions, .25 c
- Date sugar, .25 c

- Agave nectar, 2 tbsp

- Plum tomatoes, 6

What you'll do:

Let's begin by making the barbecue sauce. Add all of the barbecue sauce ingredients, minus the date sugar, to your blender and mix together until smooth and combined.

Pour all of the blended ingredients into a pot along with the date sugar. Allow the mixture to heat up until it comes to a boil. Make sure you occasionally stir it. Turn the heat down and allow it to simmer, covered, for about 15 minutes. Stir it occasionally as it cooks.

To make the sauce smoother, you can use an immersion blender at this point. With the lid off, and simmering, allow it to cook for about ten minutes more or until the water has cooked off. Let the sauce cool completely. It will thicken as it cools.

Next, add the garbanzo beans and spelt to a food processor and pulse it together for about ten to 15 seconds. Place some oil into a large skillet and add in the peppers, onions, and seasonings and sauté everything for about three to five minutes.

Stir in the pulsed ingredients, barbecue sauce, and tomato. Allow this all to simmer together for another five minutes. This is great served with some alkaline flatbread.

Native Soup

What you'll need:

- Sea salt, 2 tbsp
- Chopped red bell pepper, 1 c
- Basil, 2 tbsp
- Chopped green bell pepper, 1 c
- Oregano, 2 tsp.
- Cayenne pepper, 2 tsp.
- Gallon of spring water
- Chopped yellow squash
- Dill, 1 tsp.
- Chopped red onion
- Grapeseed oil, 2 tbsp
- Chopped butternut squash, 2 c
- Diced Roma tomatoes, 3
- Chopped zucchini
- Chopped mushrooms, 4 c
- Quinoa, 1 c – optional
- Cooked garbanzo beans, 1 lb..
- Kamut pasta, 2 to 4 c

What you'll do:

You need to make sure that you soak your garbanzo beans overnight and cook them before you mix it into your soup.

Start by adding all of the water into a large pot and let it heat up over medium. As the water heats up, clean and chop all of the vegetables and add them into the water. Mix in the seasoning and allow the soup to come up to a simmer and cook for at least an hour. Make sure that you stir the soup every few minutes. Mix in your garbanzo beans and then enjoy. You can easily freeze any leftovers of the soup for use at a later time.

Headache Salad

What you'll need:

- Cayenne pepper, to taste
- Salt, to taste
- Olive oil, 2 tbsp
- Key lime juice, 1 tbsp
- Watercress, 2 c
- Cucumber, seeded, .5

What you'll do:

Place the cucumber and watercress onto a serving plate.

Put the juice and olive oil into a small bowl and whisk until well combined.

Pour over watercress and cucumber. Sprinkle with pepper and salt. Enjoy.

Strawberry Dandelion Salad

What you'll need:

- Sea salt, to taste

- Dandelion greens, 4 c

- Key lime juice, 2 tbsp

- Sliced strawberries, 10

- Sliced red onion, 1 medium

- Grapeseed oil, 2 tbsp

What you'll do:

Place a nonstick skillet on top of the stove and warm. Add the onions and a pinch of salt. Cook while stirring until onions are slightly brown and soft.

Place one teaspoon of the lime juice into a small bowl, add in the strawberries and toss to coat.

Wash the dandelion greens and dry them with paper towels. If you prefer, you can tear or cut the greens into smaller pieces.

Once the onions are almost cooked through, add the rest of the lime juice to the onions and cook for about two minutes until onions are coated. Take off heat.

Place the strawberries, onions, and greens in a salad bowl along with all the juices. Sprinkle on some sea salt. Enjoy.

Grilled Romaine Salad

What you'll need:

- Agave syrup, 1 tbsp
- Olive oil, 4 tbsp
- Sea salt, to taste
- Onion powder, to taste
- Key lime juice, 1 tbsp
- Cayenne pepper, to taste
- Finely chopped red onion, 1 tbsp
- Chopped basil, 1 tbsp
- Romaine lettuce, 4 small heads, rinsed

What you'll do:

Cut each Romaine head in half. Place each half into a nonstick skillet cut side down. You don't need to add oil. Lettuce needs to be browned on each side. Check for doneness by lifting the lettuce up. Once all the lettuce has been browned, take off heat and let it cool on a platter.

To make the dressing: place the basil, lime juice, agave syrup, and olive oil into a small bowl. Whisk to combine. Add cayenne pepper, onion powder, and salt. Whisk again until well combined.

Place the grilled lettuce onto a serving platter and drizzle on the dressing.

Wakame Salad

What you'll need:

- Sesame oil, 1 tbsp
- Agave syrup, 1 tbsp
- Key lime juice, 1 tbsp
- Sesame seeds, 1tbsp
- Red bell pepper, 1 tbsp
- Onion powder, 1 tsp.
- Wakame stems, 2 c
- Ginger, 1 tsp.

What you'll do:

Soak the wakame stems in water for about ten minutes. Drain well.

Put the ginger, onion powder, lime juice, agave syrup, and sesame oil into a small bowl and whisk well to combine.

Put the bell pepper and wakame onto a serving platter. Drizzle on dressing and sprinkle on sesame seeds.

Roasted Vegetable and Coconut Milk Soup

What you'll need:

- Cayenne pepper, to taste

- Sea salt, to taste

- Grapeseed oil, 1 tbsp plus more for vegetables

- Coconut milk, 1 c

- Grated ginger, 1 tbsp

- Diced onion, 1 small

- Vegetable of choice, 2 c chopped

What you'll do:

Warm your oven to 350. Place your chopped vegetables onto a baking dish. Drizzle with grapeseed oil and toss to coat. Season with pepper and salt. Toss again. Place in the oven and cook 40 minutes.

While vegetables are roasting, cook the sauce. Add grapeseed oil to a skillet and warm. Add onion and let it cook for some time until it gets softened. Add ginger and cook until fragrant.

Now you need to add the coconut milk and let it come to a boil. Lessen the heat and let it continue to simmer about 30 minutes until reduced to the way you want it.

When veggies are done, carefully remove from oven.

Pour milk mixture into two bowls. Divide the vegetables evenly into the bowl. Add more seasonings if desired.

You can mash a few vegetables if you would like to.

Quinoa and Zucchini Salad

What you'll need:

- Finely chopped spring onions, 2
- Juice of one Key lime
- Olive oil, 3 tbsp
- Chickpeas, 1 can drained and rinsed
- Oregano, 1 tsp.
- Grapeseed oil, 2 tbsp
- Quinoa, .5 c
- Onion powder, 1 tsp.
- Sliced zucchini, 2 large

What you'll do:

Place the quinoa into a pot and pour in one cup of water. Allow to boil and then turn heat down and simmer until all water is absorbed about ten minutes. Cover with lid and set to the side.

Add grapeseed oil into a larger skillet and let it warm up. Put the zucchini into the pot and let the zucchini cook while you stir until they are tender but still bright green. Place into a bowl and season to taste. Put the skillet back onto the stove. Add the oregano cook while stirring until fragrant. Add this oil to the zucchini.

Add the spring onions, lime juice, olive oil, onion powder, quinoa, and chickpeas to zucchini and toss well.

Warm Quinoa and Avocado Salad

What you'll need:

- Fresh basil, handful torn into pieces

- Chickpeas, 1 can drained

- Quinoa, 1 c

- Avocados, 4 cut into quarters

What you'll do:

Cook the quinoa according to the package directions. Add the remaining ingredients to the quinoa. Toss to combine. Season to your liking.

Serve the salad warm with lime wedges and some olive oil.

Pumpkin Squash Soup

What you'll need:

- Cayenne pepper, pinch
- Sea salt, pinch
- Grapeseed oil, 1 tbsp
- Vegetable broth, 2.25 c
- Basil leaves, .5 c
- Chopped fresh ginger, small piece
- Diced onion, 1
- Coconut cream, 1 c
- Butternut squash, peeled and cubed, 4 c

What you'll do:

Place large skillet on medium heat. Put grapeseed oil in skillet and warm. Place the onion into the warmed skillet with the ginger and cook until it has softened.

Add butternut squash into the skillet and continue to cook for about ten minutes. Stirring every now and then until squash begins to soften and turn slightly brown.

Add vegetable broth and season with cayenne and salt. Allow to boil and turn heat down. Let simmer about ten minutes until squash is extremely soft.

Gently pour soup into a blender and add the cream. Place lid back onto the blender. Since the liquid is hot, you will need to hold the lid down by using a kitchen towel. Turn the blender on until it becomes smooth.

Ladle into bowls and garnish with basil leaves.

Soursop Ginger Soup

What you'll need:

- Cayenne, .25 tsp.

- Minced ginger, 1 tbsp

- Quinoa, 1 c

- Diced red pepper, 1 c

- Oregano, 1 tbsp

- Diced green peppers, 1 c

- Basil, 1 tbsp

- Diced onions, 1 c

- Sea salt, 4 tsp.

- Cubed summer squash, 1 c

- Onion powder, 3 tbsp

- Cubed zucchini, 1 c

- Cubed chayote squash, 2 c

- Chopped kale, 2 c

- Springwater, 1 gallon

- Soursop leaves, 4 to 6

What you'll do:

Rinse the soursop and rip then in half. Add them to a pot with the water. Boil the leaves for about 15 to 20 minutes.

Take the leaves out.

Add in all of the other ingredients. Add in another eight cups of water.

Mix the ingredients together. Place the lid on and cook it for 30 to 45 minutes.

Spelt Salad with Tahini

What you'll need:

Salad:

- Raisins, .25 c

- Onion, .5

- Cherry tomatoes, .25 c

- Red bell pepper

- Olive oil, 3 tbsp

- Kale, 1.5 c

- Cooked spelt, 2 c

Dressing:

- Grated ginger, 2-inch piece

- Sea salt

- Juice of a lime

- Dried oregano, 1 tbsp

- Cayenne, 1 tsp.

- Tahini, .5 c

What you'll do:

While your spelt is cooking, you can make your tahini dressing so that the flavors have time to meld together.

Start by placing the tahini, ginger, salt, lime juice, dried oregano, and cayenne in a bowl. Whisk it all together until it is well mixed. Alternatively, you can place everything in a blender and mix it up.

Next, wash the kale and remove the stems. Break the kale up into smaller pieces. You can also massage the kale with oil in order to soften it up and make it easier to eat since it won't get cooked.

Next, clean the red bell pepper and cherry tomatoes. Dice up the pepper and onion and slice the cherry tomatoes in half. Add the kale to a bowl, and top it with the oil, pepper, tomatoes, diced onion, raisins and cooked spelt. Toss everything together to coat it in the olive oil.

Pour in the dressing and toss everything together so that it is well coated. Enjoy.

Pasta and Pizza

Avocado Basil Pasta Salad

What you'll need:

- Cooked spelt pasta, 4 c
- Olive oil, .25 c
- Agave syrup, 1 tsp.
- Key lime juice, 1 tbsp
- Halved cherry tomatoes, 1 pint
- Chopped basil, 1 c
- Chopped avocado, 1

What you'll do:

Put the cooked pasta into a large bowl.

Add in the tomatoes, basil, and avocado. Toss to combine.

Put the salt, agave syrup, lime juice, and oil into a bowl. You are going to need to whisk everything vigorously in order to get everything combined.

Pour dressing on top of the pasta mixture. Now toss everything together to coat the pasta with the dressing.

Veggie Pizza

What you'll need:

- Alkaline Pizza Crust – recipe found in next section
- Brazil nut cheese
- Red bell peppers
- Green bell peppers
- Onion
- Tomatoes
- Avocado
- Mushrooms
- Oregano
- Tomato Pizza Sauce:
- Basil
- Grapeseed oil, 2 tbsp
- Oregano, 1 tsp.
- Agave, 2 tbsp
- Sea salt, 1 tsp.
- Chopped onion, 2 tbsp
- Roma tomatoes, 5
- Onion powder, 1 tsp.

- Avocado Pizza Sauce:

- Basil

- Onion powder, .5 tsp.

- Chopped onion, 2 tbsp

- Oregano, .5 tsp.

- Avocado

- Sea salt, .5 tsp.

What you'll do:

First, let's make the two pizza sauces. For the tomato sauce, start by making small x-shaped cuts on both ends of the tomatoes and then place them into some boiling water. Only let them boil for a minute.

Immediately remove the tomato from the boiling water and put it into an ice bath for 30 seconds. The skin should easily peel off. Place your prepared tomatoes into a blender along with the other tomato sauce ingredients. Blend everything together until combined.

For the avocado sauce, slice the avocado in half and take out the pit. Scrape all of the insides into your food processor. Put the remaining sauce ingredients and blend about three minutes, or until it becomes smooth.

Now let's prepare the pizza. Take your flatbread pizza crust and spread one half with the tomato sauce and the other half with the avocado sauce. Sprinkle the Brazil nut cheese over the pizza and then add what approved toppings you would like.

Make sure that your oven is warmed to 400 and then bake your pizza for 15 to 20 minutes. Enjoy.

Lasagna

What you'll need:
- Spelt lasagna sheets
- Mushrooms
- Zucchini

Tomato Sauce:
- Basil, 2 tsp.
- Cayenne pepper, .5 tsp.
- Onion powder, 1 tbsp
- Agave, 1 tbsp
- Sea salt, 2 tsp.
- Plum tomatoes, 12
- Oregano, 2 tsp.

"Meat":
- Fennel powder, 1 tsp.
- Sea salt, 1 tbsp
- Diced red, yellow, and green bell peppers, 1 c
- Basil, 2 tsp.

- Chopped onions, 1 c

- Oregano, 2 tsp.

- Cooked garbanzo beans, 1 c

- Onion powder, 2 tbsp

- Cooked spelt berries, 2 c

Cheese:

- Basil, 1 tsp.

- Hemp seeds, 1 tbsp

- Onion powder, 1 tbsp

- Springwater, 1 c

- Oregano, 1 tsp.

- Soaked brazil nuts, 2 c

- Sea salt, 1 tsp.

What you'll do:

Start by fixing the tomato sauce. Add all of the tomato sauce ingredients to your blender and mix them together until they form a sauce. Pour this into a pot and allow the sauce to begin boiling. Lower the heat down a bit and let it continue to simmer, stirring occasionally, for at least two hours, or until it has thickened up.

As this cooks, you can get the "meat" mixture together. Add the seasonings, garbanzo beans, and spelt to a food processor and mix it all together until it becomes well blended.

Add a skillet to high heat with some grapeseed oil. Add the peppers into the skillet along with the onions and let these cook for about five minutes. Mix in the garbanzo bean mixture and let everything cook for ten to 12 minutes. Everything needs to be browning up.

Now place all of the cheese mixture ingredients to your blender and mix them all together until they are well combined. If it appears too thick, add in an extra quarter cup of water slowly until it reaches the consistency you are looking for.

Reserve a cup of the tomato sauce. Add the rest of the sauce to the "meat" mixture and stir everything together. Slice up some zucchini and mushrooms.

Get a glass baking dish and add a bit of the tomato sauce to the bottom to make sure that the pasta doesn't stick to it. Lay down some pasta and top it with zucchini, "meat" mixture, cheese, and then mushrooms. Repeat this process until your lasagna has four layers. Your final layer of lasagna will be covered with the "meat" mixture and then the cheese. Pour the reserved tomato sauce around the lasagna.

Put the lasagna into the preheated oven and let it bake for 35 to 45 minutes at 350. Before you slice the lasagna, let it sit for no less than 15 minutes.

Kale and Brazil Nut Pesto with Butternut Squash

What you'll need:

Squash:

- Sea salt

- Dried sage, 1 tbsp

- Grapeseed oil, 1 tbsp

- Cubed butternut squash, 1.5 c

Pesto:

- Onion powder, 2 tsp.

- Chopped Brazil nuts, 2 tbsp

- Olive oil, 4 tbsp

- Juice of 2 limes

- Parsley, 1 tbsp

- Kale, 2 c – washed and stem removed

- Cooked quinoa, 2.5 c – to serve

What you'll do:

To start, get your oven to 400. Add the butternut squash to a bowl and drizzle in the oil. Add in the seasonings and toss everything to squash well. Pour the squash onto a baking sheet and allow it to bake for at least 30 minutes. Once it can be pierced easily with a fork, it is finished.

As the squash is cooking, add the kale, parsley, lime juice, olive oil, brazil nuts, and onion powder to your food processor. Turn the processor on and allow everything to mix together until it all comes together. The pesto may appear dry, but that's okay. This process may be loud because of the nuts.

Next, place cooked quinoa in a glass bowl and add in the pesto you just made. Mix them together until the pesto is evenly distributed throughout the quinoa. Add in the cooked butternut squash and toss everything together. You can serve this with a wedge of avocado and some basil. Enjoy.

Zoodles in Avocado Sauce

What you'll need:

- Sea salt, to taste
- Cherry tomatoes, 24 sliced
- Avocados, 2
- Key lime juice, 4 tbsp
- Walnuts, .5 c
- Water, .5 c
- Basil, 2 c
- Zucchinis, 2 large

What you'll do:

You will need to make the zoodles by either using a spiralizer or a peeler.

Place salt, avocados, lime juice, walnuts, and basil into a blender and process until creamy.

Place the zoodles into a bowl. Add tomatoes, avocado sauce, and zoodles. Toss until well coated. Enjoy.

Fried Rice

What you'll need:

- Cayenne pepper, to taste
- Sea salt, to taste
- Grapeseed oil, 1 tbsp
- Diced onion, .25
- Sliced zucchini, .5 c
- Sliced mushrooms, .5 c
- Sliced bell peppers, .5 c
- Cooked quinoa or wild rice, 1 c

What you'll do:

Place a skillet on top of stove and warm grapeseed oil. Add onion and cook until slightly browned and softened.

To the skillet, put all the other veggies and cook these for five more minutes. They should be soft but not mushy.

Add rice, stir to combine, and cook until slightly browned.

Rice and Spinach Balls

What you'll need:

- For Part One

- Juice of one key lime

- Pitted Greek olives, .33 c

- Sea salt, .75 tsp.

- Spinach leaves, 4.5 c

- Onion powder, 1 tsp.

- For Part Two

- Chickpea flour, .5 c

- Ground almonds, .5 c

- Cooked wild rice, 1.25 c

What you'll do:

Warm your oven to 360. Place all the ingredients for part one into either a food processor or a blender whichever one you have access to. Turn on the device until everything is well combined.

Add this mixture to a large bowl and add in all the ingredients for part two. Mix this together until it forms a dough. If it seems too wet, add some more flour. You can add in some cayenne pepper for taste if you would like. I don't recommend that you taste this as chickpea flour can be very bitter.

Take this mixture and scoop it out with a spoon. Roll it in between your palms until it turns into a ball. Place these onto a cookie sheet that has parchment paper on it. This should make one dozen balls. Place into the oven for 20 minutes. If you want to check for doneness, you will have to taste one of them. Be careful not to burn your mouth. If you don't taste any bitterness, they are done.

Flatbread

What you'll need:

- Sea salt, 1 tbsp
- Cayenne, .25 tsp.
- Oregano, 2 tsp.
- Springwater, .75 c
- Onion powder, 2 tsp.
- Grapeseed oil, 2 tbsp
- Basil, 2 tsp.

What you'll do:

Combine the seasonings together into the flour. Stir in the oil, and mix in a half cup of the water.

Slowly add in the rest of the water until the dough forms a ball.

Sprinkle some flour over your workspace and then knead your dough for five minutes. Divide it into six parts.

Roll the balls into four-inch circles.

Lay them out on an ungreased skillet that has been heated to medium-high. Flip it every two to three minutes, or until it is cooked through. Enjoy.

Chickpea "Tuna" Salad

What you'll need:

- Sea salt, .25 tsp.
- Dill, 1 tsp.
- Onion powder, 2 tsp.
- Nori sheet, .5
- Diced red onions, .25 c
- Alkaline mayo, .66 c
- Diced green peppers, 1/8 c
- Cooked chickpeas, 2 c

What you'll do:

Place the chickpeas in a bowl and mash them until they reached your desired consistency.

Slice the nori sheets up and mix them into the chickpeas.

Add in all of the other ingredients and stir them together.

Place the salad into the fridge for 30 minutes to an hour before you serve.

Enoki Mushroom Pasta

What you'll need:

- Sea salt
- Coconut oil, 1 tbsp
- Onions
- Bell pepper
- Handful of plum tomatoes
- Enoki mushrooms, 10.5 oz
- Butternut squash, 2 round slices

What you'll do:

Start by getting your butternut squash ready. Peel the squash and then dice it up. Place the squash into a pot and let it begin boiling, cooking until soft. Once they are soft, pour out the water and then mash then into a paste.

Juice your tomatoes and then mix this into your squash. This will thin the squash paste out a bit and will add more flavor. If you want, you can mix in some Irish moss jelly at this point, but you don't have to.

Mix in the onion, bell pepper, and mushrooms. Allow this all to simmer together for two to five minutes.

Then add in some salt to taste. Allow this to cool for five to ten minutes and then stir in the coconut oil. The coconut oil will create a really nice rich flavor. Enjoy.

Pasta with Walnut Pesto

What you'll need:

- Walnuts, .5 c
- Juice of a lime
- Sea salt
- Fresh basil, 3 c
- Avocado
- Spelt pasta, .5 c

What you'll do:

To start, add the basil, avocado, walnuts, lime juice, and salt to a food processor. Mix all of the ingredients together until they form a smooth sauce.

Next, cook your spelt pasta according to the directions on the packaging. Once cooked, drain, and pour into a bowl. Pour in the pesto and mix everything together. At this point, you can mix in some extra Dr. Sebi approved ingredients like chopped olives, chopped tomatoes, and torn basil. Enjoy.

Vegetable Alfredo

What you'll need:

- Grapeseed oil
- Sea salt
- Oregano
- Basil
- An orange bell pepper
- Onion powder
- A zucchini
- Cayenne
- An onion
- A red bell pepper
- A summer squash
- A container of mushrooms
- Spelt tortiglioni pasta, 10 oz bag
- Sauce:
- Grapeseed oil, 2 tsp.
- Springwater, 1.5 c
- Hemp milk, 1.5 c
- Cayenne, .5 tsp.

- Juice of .5 a lime

- Onion powder, 1 tsp.

- Soaked brazil nuts, 1 lb..

- Sea salt, 2 tsp.

What you'll do:

Start by making the sauce. Add everything except for the spring water into your food processor. Add in a half of a cup of water and blend everything together for almost two minutes. Continue to pour in another half of a cup of water and blend until it reaches the consistency that you like. You can use the sauce for just about anything.

Next, boil the pasta like the directions tell you to on the packaging and then drain well. While you are cooking the pasta, chop up your vegetables.

Add a little bit of oil to the skillet and in a little bit of each of the vegetables. Mix in a teaspoon of the herbs and seasonings. Lightly cook these veggies for a few minutes.

Put the past in with the vegetables and pour some cheese sauce in. Stir everything together and sauté for another minute. Enjoy.

Mushroom Stroganoff

What you'll need:

- Basil, 1 tsp.

- Water, 2 c

- Sea salt, to taste

- Kale, 1 c

- Cayenne pepper, .5 tsp.

- Onion, 1

- Red bell pepper. 1

- Oregano, 1 tsp.

- Chickpea flour, .5 c

- Onion powder, 1 tsp.

- Brazil nuts, .5 c

- Savory, 1 tsp.

- Portobello mushrooms, 3 c

- Spelt pasta, 1 lb.

What you'll do:

You need to fix the pasta the way the package tells you to. Drain the pasta well and leave it in cold water so it won't stick together.

Place one cup of water, cayenne, onion powder, salt, and Brazil nuts into a blender. Process until creamy and smooth.

Dice the onion, red bell pepper, and mushrooms. Place in a skillet. Add seasoning to your liking and sauté in two tablespoons water until tender.

Add in the chickpea flour and more water and whisk until you have a gravy-like consistency. You can add more flour or water as you need to.

Cut the kale into bite-size pieces. Add to the gravy and stir to coat. Simmer until kale has been cooked through. This will take about 15 minutes.

Give everything a taste and add any seasonings if you need to.

Drain the pasta and put it in the gravy. Stir well to coat pasta.

Serve and enjoy.

Walnut Kale Pasta

What you'll need:

- Cayenne pepper, to taste
- Sea salt, to taste
- Avocado oil, 2 tbsp
- Chopped onion, 1 small
- Walnut flakes, .33 c
- Spelt pasta, 1.5 c
- Kale, 3 c

What you'll do:

Begin by fixing the pasta the way the package tells you to. It still needs to be "al dente."

Wash the kale and chop into bite-size pieces.

Put the avocado oil in a large skillet and slowly heat it up then add the onion. Allow the onion to cook until it has softened and turned a translucent color now put the kale into the skillet and stir to combine with onions. Add some water and cook until kale is wilted.

In another dry skillet, add the walnut flakes and toast gently.

Once the kale is wilted, add pasta, and stir well to combine.

Sprinkle with walnut flakes and season to taste.

Tomato Pasta

What you'll need:

- Spelt pasta, 1 lb.
- Olive oil, 2 tbsp
- Bell pepper, 1
- Zucchini, 1 medium
- Onion, 1 large
- Chickpeas, 1 15 oz can
- Chopped tomatoes, 5

What you'll do:

Start by fixing the pasta the way the package tells you to.

Wash and chop the zucchini, onion, bell pepper, and tomatoes. Add to a skillet along with some water.

"Steam fry" the vegetables until tender.

Drain and rinse the chickpeas. Put them in the tomato mixture and cook five minutes or until they have been warmed through.

Drain the pasta and divide it evenly into plates. Divide the sauce evenly and pour on the pasta. If you want the extra flavor, you can drizzle some olive oil on top and enjoy.

Spicy Sesame Ginger Noodle Bowl

What you'll need:

- Spelt angel hair pasta, 8 oz

- Sesame oil, 2 tbsp

- Peeled and chopped cucumber, 1

- Onion powder, 1 tsp.

- Walnut butter, 1 tbsp

- Tahini, 1 tbsp

- Juice of one key lime

- Grated ginger, 1 tbsp

- Sea salt, to taste

- Cayenne pepper, to taste

What you'll do:

Fix the pasta as per the directions on the package. Drain and rinse with cool water. Leave in colander while you make the dressing.

Add the onion powder, ginger, lime juice, sesame oil, tahini, walnut butter, cayenne, salt, and cucumber to a small bowl. Whisk until walnut butter and tahini are incorporated together. Taste and adjust seasonings if needed.

Place pasta in a large bowl and pour dressing over the top. Toss to coat.

You may garnish with black sesame seeds and lime wedges if desired.

Zucchini Tomato Pasta

What you'll need:

- Key lime wedges, 2
- Zucchini, 2 medium
- Sea salt, to taste
- Basil, 1 tsp.
- Chopped tomatoes, 2
- Oregano, 1 tsp.
- Chopped onion, 1 medium
- Avocado oil, 2 tsp.

What you'll do:

Begin by warming some avocado oil in a skillet. Add the onion to the skillet and let the onion cook until it has softened. Add in salt, oregano, basil, and tomatoes. Stir well and continue cooking until the tomatoes are soft and the ingredients have cooked together. This will take about four minutes.

Using either a spiralizer or peeled, turn the zucchini into noodles. Divide them equally between two plates. Add one lime wedge to each plate.

If you want your zucchini heated through, you can add it to the sauce for a minute. Cooking the zucchini for too long will lose some of its nutrients.

When ready to eat, squeeze the lime over the pasta and enjoy.

Creamy Mushroom Pasta

What you'll need:

- Cayenne pepper, to taste

- Coconut milk, 3 c

- Sea salt, to taste

- Chickpea Flour, 3 tbsp

- Mixed mushrooms, 8 c

- Chopped onion, 1 medium

- Avocado oil, .25 c

- Spelt pasta, 1 lb.

What you'll do:

In a large pasta pot, pour eight cups water and add a large handful of sea salt. Cook the pasta like the package states. When done, drain.

While the pasta cooks, you can get the sauce ready.

Warm the avocado oil in a skillet. Place the onions, mushroom, and a pinch of salt. Cook while occasionally stirring until mushrooms have softened and are slightly browned. This will take about 15 minutes. Turn the heat down after five minutes have passed.

Sprinkle the flour over the mushroom mixture and stir well. Make sure everything is covered with the flour. Let this cook for about one minute. You will need to turn your heat back up.

Add in one cup of the coconut milk while constantly stirring and simmer for one minute. Break up any clumps that might have formed.

Once it is totally smooth and has thickened a bit, add the rest of the coconut milk. Add some cayenne for your taste and bring the liquid to a simmer while constantly stirring.

Continue cooking until the sauce has thickened one more time.

Take off heat. Taste and adjust seasonings if needed.

Place the cooked pasta into the sauce. Toss well to coat everything.

Divide into serving plates and enjoy.

Creamy Kamut Pasta

What you'll need:

Pasta:

- Onion powder, 1 tsp.

- Grapeseed oil, 2 tbsp

- Kamut spirals, 12 oz

- Sea salt, 1 tsp.

- Springwater, 8 c

- Dried tarragon, 1 tbsp

Sauce:

- Kale, 2 c

- Onion powder, 2 tsp.

- Chopped plum tomatoes, 3

- Basil, 1 tsp.

- Coconut milk, 1 15 oz can

- Oregano, 1 tsp.

- Springwater, 2 c

- Tarragon, 1 tbsp

- Chickpea flour, .25 c

- Cayenne pepper, .25 tsp. + .5 tsp. more

- Sea salt, .25 tsp. + .5 tsp. more

- Sliced baby bella mushrooms, 1 lb.

- Chopped onion, .5 medium

- Grapeseed oil, 2 tbsp, divided

What you'll do:

For Pasta

Add the water to a large pasta pot. Allow to boil and add a handful of salt.

When the water is boiling, add the pasta. Cook for ten minutes. When pasta is done, drain and place into a bowl. Sit to the side.

Add onion powder, sea salt, tarragon, and grapeseed oil to a small bowl. Whisk together and pour over warm pasta. Toss to coat. Taste and adjust seasonings if needed.

For Sauce

Add one tablespoon grapeseed oil to the pot you used to cook the pasta. Put the pot on medium heat and let the oil warm.

Add the sliced mushrooms and chopped onions to warmed oil. Cook the vegetables until they have become soft. Put .25 teaspoon cayenne and .25 teaspoon salt to the vegetables. Stir well.

Add one tablespoon grapeseed oil and the chickpea flour. Stir to mix the flour and oil into the vegetables for about one minute. Make sure all the vegetables are covered with flour.

Add in .5 teaspoon cayenne pepper, .5 teaspoon salt, onion powder, basil, oregano, tarragon, coconut milk, and water. Stir well to combine and let simmer about 20 minutes until sauce begins to thicken.

Once 20 minutes are up, add kale, tomatoes, and pasta. Stir until kale has been reduced. Take off heat. If your sauce is still a bit liquid, the sauce will thicken as it stands for a bit.

Serve and enjoy.

If you are prepping this for meals to be eaten later, just divide it evenly into six containers. This will keep in the fridge for about four days. Never store at room temperature. This recipe doesn't freeze well.

Chicken and Waffles

What you'll need:

Waffles:

- Sea salt, .25 tsp.

- Sea moss gel, 2 tsp. – optional

- Grapeseed oil, 3 tbsp

- Agave nectar, .25 c

- Oregano, 1 tsp.

- Springwater, 1 c

- Hemp milk, 1 c

- Basil, 1 tsp.

- Spelt Flour, 2 c

Mushroom "Chicken":

- Cayenne pepper, .5 tsp.

- Sea salt, .5 tsp.

- Waffle batter, .75 c

- Onion powder, 2 tsp.

- Garbanzo bean flour, .75 c

- Oyster mushrooms, 1 to 2 bunches

What you'll do:

To start, add the waffle ingredients along with a half of a cup of water to a large bowl and stir everything together until it is well combined. If it is too thick, you can mix in a little more water.

Heat up your waffle maker and then brush it with some grapeseed oil. Reserve ¾ of a cup of the batter for the chicken. Pour some of the batter into your waffle maker and cook it following the instructions for your waffle maker. Once done, set aside and keep warm. Continue to do this until you have used up the rest of the batter.

For the chicken, take the stem off of the mushrooms and clean them. Add the garbanzo bean flour and half of each of the seasonings into a lidded container. Stir them together. Add the mushrooms and place the lid on the bowl and toss everything together so that the mushrooms are well coated.

Add the rest of the seasonings to your reserved waffle batter. Mix in some water to thin it out slightly. Add the mushrooms to the batter, coating them completely. Place a few tablespoons oil into a skillet and heat up. Put the mushrooms in the skillet and cook for about three to four minutes, flipping them halfway through. Alternatively, you can bake them for 15 to 20 minutes at 400.

To serve, place a couple of pieces of chicken on top of a waffle and then drizzle them with some agave and sprinkle it with some crushed red pepper. Enjoy.

Quiche

What you'll need:

Crust:

- Onion powder, 1 tsp.
- Sea salt, 1 tsp.
- Springwater, 1 c
- Basil, 1 tsp.
- Spelt Flour, 1 c
- Oregano, 1 tsp.

Filling:

- Cayenne pepper, .25 tsp.
- Sea moss gel, 1 tbsp – optional
- Sea salt, 1 tsp.
- Green, yellow, and red pepper, .5 c
- Oregano, 1 tsp.
- Onion, .5 c
- Aquafaba, .75 c
- Basil, 1 tsp.
- Hemp milk, .75 c

- Onion powder, 1 tbsp

- Brazil nut cheese, 1 c

- Chopped kale, 1 c

- Sliced mushrooms, 2 c

- Garbanzo bean flour, 1 c

What you'll do:

To make the crust, add the seasonings and the flour to a bowl and mix together. Add in a quarter cup of water in at a time, stirring until completely mixed each time. Once it starts to form a ball, it is finished. If you get it too wet, add in more flour.

Flour your workspace and sprinkle some on your dough. Roll the dough out so that it will fit into a pie pan. You may need to apply more flour so that it doesn't stick.

Brush some grapeseed oil onto a pie plate and ease the crust into the plate. Press the dough down into the pan and trim off the excess edges.

To make the filling, add the seasonings, sea moss gel, aquafaba, milk, and flour to a blender and mix together until it is well blended.

Make sure that you have your oven set to 350. Mix together the kale, peppers, onions, and mushrooms together in a big bowl.

Pour the veggies into your pie plate, pour in the brazil nut cheese, and then pour the filling mixture over everything. Place some foil over the pie plate and then bake the quiche for 55 to 65 minutes. Take the foil off during the last ten minutes of baking.

Let the quiche cool slightly before you slice into it. Enjoy.

Macaroni and Cheese

What you'll need:

- Hemp milk, 1 c

- Juice of a .5 of a lime

- Ground annatto, .5 tsp.

- Grapeseed oil, 2 tsp.

- Onion powder, 2 tsp.

- Garbanzo bean flour, .25 c

- Sea salt, 1 tsp.

- Soaked brazil nuts, .5 lb.

- Springwater, 1 c

- Box of Kamut spirals, 12 oz

What you'll do:

Begin by cooking your Kamut spirals according to the directions on the box.

Make sure that your oven is warmed to 350. Next, we'll make the brazil nut sauce. Add the brazil nuts and all of the other ingredients into your blender and mix them together for about three minutes, or until creamy.

Brush a baking dish with some grapeseed oil. Add the pasta to the baking dish and drizzle with some more oil. Pour the brazil nut sauce over the sauce and then bake it for 30 minutes.

If you would like a crispy top, you can broil the macaroni for five minutes. Enjoy.

Ravioli

What you'll need:

Filling:

- Crushed red pepper flakes, .5 tsp.
- Cayenne pepper, .5 tsp.
- Dill, 2 tsp.
- Fennel seeds, 2 tsp.
- Thyme, 2 tsp.
- Roma tomato
- Sea salt, 1 tsp.
- Diced onion, .33 c
- Ginger, 1 tsp.
- Diced red bell pepper, .33 c
- Oregano, 2 tsp.
- Diced green bell pepper, .33 c
- Basil, 2 tsp.
- Chopped kale, 1 c
- Onion powder, 1 tbsp
- Garbanzo bean flour, 1 c
- Sliced mushrooms, 2 c

Dough:

- Basil, .5 tsp.

- Springwater, .75 c

- Oregano, .5 tsp.

- Garbanzo bean flour, .5 c

- Sea salt, 1 tsp.

- Spelt Flour, 1.5 c

Cheese:

- Oregano, .5 tsp.

- Sea salt, 1 tsp.

- Springwater, .5 c

- Onion powder, 2 tsp.

- Soaked brazil nuts, .5 c

- Cayenne, .5 tsp.

What you'll do:

Start by fixing the filling. Add the filling ingredients, minus the garbanzo bean flour, to your food processor, and mix everything together for about 30 seconds. Now you can mix the flour in until everything is well blended.

Using a cast-iron skillet, warm some grapeseed oil and then spread the ravioli filling into the skillet. Cook this for about three to four minutes. Flip the filling over and continue to cook it for another three to four minutes.

Break the filling apart and then cook it for a few more minutes. Scoop it out and put it in a bowl. Set this aside.

Now, place all of the cheese ingredients into a blender and process it all together until it is smooth. You can add extra spring water if you find that it is too thick. Pour the cheese out another bowl.

Next, add all of the dry ingredients for the dough into your food processor. Mix them together for about ten seconds and then slowly start to pour some water in as it blends until it starts to form a ball. If by chance, you don't own a food processor, you could do this part using your hands by kneading the ingredients together until it forms a ball.

Now you need to take about one-quarter of the dough and form it into a ball by rolling it between your palms. Flour your work surface and then roll the dough out. You can add more flour if it starts to stick.

Mix together the filling mixture and the cheese mixture. Place spoonfuls of the mixture on one half of the dough, placing them about a half-inch apart.

Fold the dough over the filling and press it down around the filling. Using a pastry cutter, cut the ravioli out and make sure each of the ravioli is sealed. You can, at this point, freeze the ravioli for later use.

Add some spring water to a pot along with a little bit of sea salt and oil. Allow this mixture to come up to a boil and add in the ravioli. Let the ravioli cook for four to six minutes.

Once the ravioli is cooked, remove it from the water with a strainer and allow it to cool slightly before serving. This goes well with some alkaline tomato sauce.

Wraps and Sandwiches

Nori-Burritos

What you'll need:

- Sesame seeds
- Tahini, 1 tbsp
- Sprouted hemp seeds, handful
- Dandelion greens or amaranth, handful
- Zucchini, 1 small, cut into rounds
- Nori seaweed, 4 sheets
- Sliced mango, .5
- Cucumber, seeded, sliced
- Sliced avocado

What you'll do:

Put the Nori sheets onto a cutting board. Make sure the shiny side is facing the cutting board.

Place all the ingredients onto the Nori in whatever arrangement you would like. Leave about one inch uncovered on the right side of the Nori.

Use both hands and begin folding the Nori from the side closest to you. Roll it over the filling.

Slice into two-inch thick slices and sprinkle over sesame seeds.

Grilled Zucchini and Hummus Wrap

What you'll need:

- Cayenne pepper, to taste
- Sea salt, to taste
- Grapeseed oil, 1 tbsp
- Spelt flour tortillas, 2
- Hummus, 4 tbsp
- Wild arugula or romaine lettuce, 1 c
- Red onion, .25 sliced
- Sliced plum tomato, 1
- Zucchini, ends removed and sliced, 1

What you'll do:

Place a skillet over medium heat and warm.

Place the zucchini into a bowl and sprinkle over the grapeseed oil. Toss to coat. Add cayenne pepper and salt and toss again.

Put coated zucchini in the skillet and cook for three minutes. Gently turn over and cook an additional two minutes. Set aside.

Put the tortillas into the same skillet for about one minute until slightly browned but still pliable. Turnover and warm up the other side. Take out of skillet and place on cutting board.

To assemble wraps: place two tablespoons hummus onto each wrap. Spread to cover. Add the sliced tomatoes, onion, greens, and zucchini on top of the hummus.

Roll each wrap, slice in half, enjoy.

Portobello Burgers

What you'll need:

- Purslane, 1 c
- Oregano, 1 tsp.
- Sliced avocado, 1
- Onion powder, 1 tsp.
- Sliced tomato, 1
- Cayenne pepper, .5 tsp.
- Olive oil, 3 tbsp
- Portobello mushroom caps, 2 large
- Basil, 2 tsp.

What you'll do:

Heat your oven to 425.

Take the stem off each Portobello and scrape out the "ribs." Slice each cap in half as if you are making a "bun."

Place the cayenne pepper, oregano, basil, onion powder, and olive oil into a small bowl. Whisk well to combine.

Place foil onto a baking sheet and brush on some grapeseed oil. Put mushroom caps onto the prepared baking sheet.

Spoon one tablespoon of the marinade onto each mushroom and let it sit for ten minutes.

Place into preheated oven and cook for ten minutes.

Carefully remove from oven and turn over each mushroom. Place back into the oven and cook an additional ten minutes.

Put the "bottom" of the mushroom onto a plate. Add desired toppings and top with "top" part of mushroom. Enjoy.

Veggie Fajitas

What you'll need:

- Avocado
- Cayenne pepper, to taste
- Onion powder, to taste
- Wild rice tortillas, 6
- Grapeseed oil, 1 tbsp
- Juice of .5 key lime
- Thinly sliced onion, 1
- Bell peppers, 2
- Large Portobello mushrooms, 3

What you'll do:

Wipe mushrooms with damp cloth if needed. Remove stems and clean out gills. Cut thickly into slices.

Cut the top off the bell peppers and carefully cut out the ribs and seeds and slice into thin strips.

Warm the grapeseed oil in a skillet. Put the onions along with the peppers and cook for two minutes until just getting soft.

Add seasonings and mushrooms. Stir well to combine. Continue to cook until vegetables are to desired tenderness.

Warm up the tortillas and then spoon vegetable mixture into each tortilla. Serve with lime juice and avocado.

Spelt Bread

What you'll need:

- Springwater, .75 to 1 c
- Coconut milk, .5 c
- Avocado oil, 3 tbsp
- Baking soda, 1 tsp.
- Agave nectar, 1 tbsp
- Spelt Flour, 4 c + .5 c more
- Sea salt, 1.5 tsp.

What you'll do:

You need to warm your oven to 375.

Using a large bowl, put the baking soda, salt, and flour inside. Using a whisk, and mix these well.

Add in .75 cups of the water, coconut milk, oil, and mix until combined. This mixture needs to be soft but still hold together in one clump. If it feels too stiff, add one tablespoon of water until it will easily stir. If it is too wet and won't hold together, add a tablespoon of flour, and mix after each spoonful until the dough will hold together.

Sprinkle your surface with more flour and place the dough onto the flour. Roll it around carefully to coat with the flour. Gently knead for three minutes adding small amounts of flour until the dough becomes a unified ball that will spring back when you poke it with your finger.

Place parchment paper into a normal loaf pan across the width. Lightly grease the loaf pan with avocado oil. Put the dough inside the loaf pan and pat it down so that it is in one even layer. Using a sharp knife, score the top of the loaf lengthwise. Place it into the oven for 45 minutes.

When time is done, remove from oven and check for doneness by inserting an object into the center of the bread. If, when the object is taken out, it is clean, the bread is done. If not, put it back into the oven for another ten minutes.

Allow the loaf to cool completely in the pan before you slice it.

This bread is best served toasted. This will crisp the bread and makes it taste even better. This is great topped with avocado and sprinkled with lime juice and cayenne.

Chickpea Burger

What you'll need:

- Grapeseed oil

- Sea salt, 2 tsp.

- Springwater, .25 to .5 c

- Cayenne powder, .5 tsp.

- Ginger powder, .5 tsp.

- Dill, 1 tsp.

- Onion powder, 2 tsp.

- Diced plum tomatoes, 1

- Oregano, 2 tsp.

- Diced kale, .5 c

- Basil, 2 tsp.

- Diced green peppers, .5 c

- Chopped onion, .5 c

- Chickpea flour, 1 c

What you'll do:

Find a bowl large enough to hold all of the above ingredients. Put all of these into the bowl except the flour. Mix everything well. Place all the vegetables and spices into a large bowl. Mix well. Now put the flour in and mix again.

Slowly add water while stirring until the mixture can be formed easily into a patty. If the mixture is too thin, add more flour.

Place grapeseed oil into large skillet and warm. Place patties into skillet and cook until browned on each side.

Serve on alkaline flatbread with favorite allowed toppings.

Mushroom Cheese Steak

What you'll need:

Mushrooms:

- Savory, 1 tsp.

- Grapeseed oil, 1 tbsp

- Red bell pepper, 1 c

- Thyme, 1 tsp.

- Green bell pepper, 1 c

- Oregano, 1 tsp.

- Sliced onion, 1 c

- Smoked sea salt, 1 tsp.

- Portabella mushroom caps, 4

- Onion powder, 1 tbsp

Cheese:

- Basil, .5 tsp.

- Sea salt, .5 tsp.

- Cayenne, .5 tsp.

- Hemp seeds, 1.5 tsp.

- Springwater, .33 to .5 c

- Oregano, .5 tsp.

- Soaked brazil nuts, .75 c

- Onion powder, 1.5 tsp.

What you'll do:

Take the mushrooms and slice them very thinly.

Beat all of the seasonings together with just enough olive oil to make a marinade.

Add the mushrooms into the marinade and let them rest for 30 minutes. Stir them halfway through.

As those marinate, add all of the ingredients for the cheese into a blender. Turn the blender on until all ingredients are smooth.

Pour the grapeseed oil into a skillet and add the peppers and onions. Sauté them for three to five minutes. Mix in the mushrooms and sauté for another five minutes. Serve topped with the cheese.

Enjoy as-is, or on a flatbread.

Squash Falafels

What you'll need:

- Grapeseed oil, 1 tbsp
- Sea salt
- Chickpea flour, .5 c
- Cayenne pepper, 1 tbsp
- Small white onion
- Dried oregano, 2 tbsp
- Fresh coriander, 3 tbsp
- Fresh parsley, 3 tbsp
- Tahini, 1 tbsp
- Cooked chickpeas, 3 c
- Dried dill, 2 tbsp
- Butternut squash, 1c
- Onion powder, 2 tbsp
- Dressing:
- Water, .25 c
- Tahini, 2 tbsp
- Dried dill, 1 tsp.
- Juice of a lime

- Dried oregano, 1 tsp.

- Sea salt

- Cayenne pepper, .5 tsp.

What you'll do:

Start out by steaming your butternut squash for at least 20 minutes. You can check for softness by piercing a piece with a fork. If the fork goes in easily, it is done.

Once the butternut squash is prepared, add the squash, chickpeas, tahini, parsley, coriander, onion powder, dill, oregano, cayenne, onion, chickpea flour, salt, and grapeseed oil to a food processor. Mix it all together until it forms a moist dough.

Using an ice cream scooper, scoop out the falafel mixture on a parchment-lined cookie sheet. Once you have scooped out all of the dough, all the falafels to bake for 20 minutes and 400.

As the falafels cook, add all of the dressing recipes to a bowl and mix together using a whisk or fork. You can adjust the amount of water depending on how thin you want it to be.

Once everything is done, you can serve the falafels on homemade flatbread along with a drizzle of the dressing. Enjoy.

Home Fries

What you'll need:

- Grapeseed oil
- Cayenne pepper, .5 tsp.
- Diced plum tomato
- Oregano, 1 tsp.
- Diced green bell pepper, .25 c
- Sea salt, 1 tsp.
- Diced onion, .25 c
- Green bananas, 3

What you'll do:

To get the best results with this recipe, make sure that your bananas still have green skin. Green skinned bananas should be firm, and they tend to taste a lot like potatoes when they are cooked. The more yellow the skin is, the more it will taste like banana and the softer they will become when cooked.

Begin by chopping the end off of each of the bananas and then slice them in half. Then slice each of the halves lengthwise. Carefully wedge your finger between the banana and the skin and pull the skin off.

Slice the bananas thinly and then place it in a bowl. Pour the oil over them and gently toss them to coat. Add all of the seasonings and toss them all together. Let this rest for about five to ten minutes.

Add about two tablespoons of oil into a large skillet and let it heat up to medium. Add in the home fries. Keep them spread evenly across the pan. Add in the tomatoes, peppers, and onions.

Continue to cook everything for five to seven minutes before you start flipping the food. Flip them, and then let them cook for another five minutes, stirring occasionally.

You can enjoy these as they are or with some alkaline ketchup.

Chicken Tenders

What you'll need:

Sage, 2 tsp.

- Grapeseed oil

- Allspice, 1 tsp.

- Sea salt, 2 tsp.

- Basil, 2 tsp.

- Oregano, 2 tsp.

- Spelt Flour, 1.5 c

- Cayenne pepper, 1 tsp.

- Aquafaba or Springwater, 1.5 c

- Ginger powder, 2 tsp.

- Portabella mushrooms, 2 to 6

- Onion powder, 2 tsp.

What you'll do:

The aquafaba mentioned above is simply the water that comes off of garbanzo beans.

To start, slice the mushroom caps into half-inch slices and then lay them in a large bowl. You can use the mushroom stems to make "chicken" nuggets. Add half of each of the seasonings, aquafaba, and some of the oil into the container and mix everything together so that the mushrooms are coated. Let this sit and marinate for about an hour. Mix together the remaining seasonings and the flour together. Coat all of the mushroom pieces in the flour mixture.

Make sure that you have your oven to 400. Brush some oil on a baking sheet a lay the mushroom pieces across the baking sheet. Allow them to bake for 15 minutes, flip them over, and then let them cook for another 15 minutes, or until they are crispy. Enjoy them as is, or place them on some Dr. Sebi approved bread.

Hot Dogs

What you'll need:

- Grapeseed oil
- Crushed red pepper, .5 tsp. – optional
- Fennel, .5 tsp.
- Dill, .5 tsp.
- Ginger, .5 tsp.
- Coriander, 1 tsp.
- Diced shallots, .25 c
- Diced onion, .33 c
- Onion powder, 1 tbsp
- Diced green bell pepper, .33 c
- Smoked sea salt, 2 tsp.
- Aquafaba, .5 c
- Spelt Flour, 1 c
- Garbanzo beans, 1 c

What you'll do:

Begin by heating up a skillet with some grapeseed oil and add in the vegetables and garbanzo beans. Sauté everything together for about five minutes until they are soft.

Add the vegetables into a food processor along with all of the other ingredients. Mix them all together until they are well blended. This is your hot dog mixture.

You can either use your hands or a hot dog mold for the next step. Take the mixture and mash it into a hot dog mold, or you can roll it into a hot dog shape using your hands. Wrap the hot dogs in some parchment paper.

Place a steamer basket inside a pot. Pour some water into the pot and boil the water. Lay the hot dogs on the steamer and let them steam for around 30 to 40 minutes. After they are done steaming, take the parchment paper off of them, or take them out of the mold.

To brown up the hot dogs, add some grapeseed oil to a skillet and brown for five to ten minutes. Enjoy your hot dogs on some Dr. Sebi approved hot dog buns with some alkaline ketchup.

Spring Rolls

What you'll need:

Kale Filling:

- Grapeseed oil, 2 tsp.
- Thinly sliced red bell pepper, .5
- Onion powder, 1 tsp.
- Sliced onion, .5 c
- Kale, 3 c
- Sea salt, 1 tsp.
- Avocado Filling:
- Sea salt, .5 tsp.
- Diced green bell peppers, 2 tbsp
- Onion powder, 1 tsp.
- Diced red bell onion, 2 tbsp
- Lime juice, 1 tsp.
- Avocado

Spring Rolls:

- Springwater, .5 c
- Grapeseed oil, .33 c

- Onion powder, 1 tsp.

- Spelt Flour, 2 c

- Sea salt, 1 tsp.

What you'll do:

Let's start by making the spring rolls. Add the seasonings and the flour to your food processor and mix everything together for about ten seconds. Slowly add in the grapeseed oil as it is mixing.

Slowly add in the water as it is mixing until a dough ball forms. Sprinkle your work surface with some flour and lay out the dough. Knead the dough until it comes together and then separate it out into five parts, as equal as you can.

Roll each of the sections out into a thin circle. Using a food scraper, cut out a six-inch square. Roll the cut off dough into a ball and continue to do this. Continue to make these squares until you have used up all of the dough. As you do this, place parchment paper between the dough so it doesn't stick.

Once the dough has been prepared, move onto getting the filling mixed together. For the kale filling, heat up a skillet and sauté everything together for about five to seven minutes, or until the veggies become tender.

For the avocado filling, slice the avocado in half, remove the pit, and then scoop out the filling. Add in all of the other ingredients and then mash everything together.

To assemble, brush the edges and corners of the dough with aquafaba before you roll it up so that it sticks together.

Add two to three tablespoons of a filling into the center of the dough. Pull the bottom corner up and over the filling and then fold in the right and left sides into the middle, and then roll up towards the top corner. You want it tight enough so that the filling doesn't fall out.

In a lightly greased skillet, place the egg roll in the pan and cook for about a minute on both sides. Once the sides are done, fry on the very ends of the roll. Enjoy.

Cereals

Hummus

What you'll need:

- Sea salt, to taste
- Onion powder, dash
- Juice of one key lime
- Tahini butter, .33 c
- Olive oil, 2 tbsp
- Cooked chickpeas, 1 c

What you'll do:

You will need to put the ingredients listed above into your blender. Turn the blender on and leave it on until creamy and smooth.

Crunchy Hummus

What you'll need:

- Red onion, .5

- Fresh coriander, 2 tbsp

- Cherry tomatoes, .25 c

- Red bell pepper, .5

- Dulse flakes, 1 tbsp

- Juice of a lime

- Sea salt

- Olive oil, 3 tbsp

- Tahini, 2 tbsp

- Warm chickpeas, 1 c

What you'll do:

Start by warming your chickpeas. You can do this in a couple of different ways. You can place them on a baking sheet in an oven that has been heated to 250. Simply keep an eye on them, stirring them every five minutes or so until lightly warmed. You can also do this in a skillet. Stir the chickpeas every few minutes to make sure they don't burn until they are lightly warmed.

Then add your warmed chickpeas to a bowl along with the tahini, sea salt, and lime. With a fork, mash the chickpeas and ingredients together until it forms a paste. It doesn't have to be perfectly smooth.

Add in the chopped onion, cherry tomatoes, bell pepper, dulse flakes, and olive oil. Mix everything together until it is well combined. Enjoy this hummus on a couple of slices of organic spelt bread.

Vegetable Quinoa

What you'll need:

- Cayenne, .5 tsp.

- Grapeseed oil, 2 tbsp

- Diced plum tomato

- Oregano, 1 tsp.

- Diced red onion, .5 c

- Basil, 1 tsp.

- Springwater, .5 c

- Onion powder, 1 tsp.

- Diced yellow bell pepper, .25 c

- Sea salt, 2 tsp.

- Diced green bell pepper, .25 c

- Diced red bell pepper, .25

- Chipped zucchini, 1 c

- Cooked quinoa, 4 c

What you'll do:

Add your oil into a skillet. Add in the vegetables and the seasonings. Cook them for five to ten minutes.

Add quinoa and water. Stir well and cook for five minutes more. Enjoy.

Kamut Cereal

What you'll need:

- Sea salt
- Oregano
- Onion powder
- Cayenne
- Spring water, 2 c
- Kamut, 1 c

What you'll do:

Pour the water into a pot and add in the sea salt. Leave alone until it begins to boil. Add a cup of the Kamut berries to a food processor and grind them up until they start to look like grits.

Add the Kamut into the boiling water. Constantly stir the Kamut as it is cooking. You can add more spring water when you need to in order to reach your desired consistency.

You can add in whatever seasoning you would like to and enjoy.

Kamut Puff Cereal

What you'll need:

- Agave nectar

- Kamut puffs, 6 oz bag

What you'll do:

This is a Dr. Sebi approved version of the family favorite corn puffs.

Begin by spreading the Kamut puffs over a baking sheet. Drizzle them with the agave nectar and stir to coat. Make sure that your oven is set to 350 and cook the puffs for 11 minutes.

Allow the puffs to cool for 10 to 15 minutes. Break the puffs up and keep them stored in an airtight container. Enjoy them in a bowl of coconut milk.

Teff Porridge

What you'll need:

- Blueberries – optional

- Agave – optional

- Sea salt, pinch

- Springwater, 2 c

- Teff grain, .5 c

What you'll do:

Start by adding the water to a pot and letting come up to a boil. Add in the sea salt. Once the water has started to boil, slowly pour in the teff grain as you stir the water.

Place the lid onto the pot and turn the heat down so that the teff simmers for about 15 minutes. Serve the teff with a drizzle of the agave and some blueberries. If you would prefer, you can choose a different Dr. Sebi approved fruit to top your teff with. Enjoy.

Quinoa Cereal

What you'll need:

- Your favorite approved fruits, .33 c

- Your favorite approved milk, .5 to 1 c

- Warmed pre-cooked quinoa, .5 c

- Agave nectar or date sugar – optional

- Toasted nuts, coconut flakes, favorite spices - optional

What you'll do:

This is a quick and easy breakfast to do when you have some leftover quinoa from last night's dinner.

All you have to do is warm up the quinoa, mix in a bit of your favorite milk, and top with your favorite and other add-ins that you would like. Enjoy.

Desserts

Zucchini Bread Pancakes

What you'll need:

- Grapeseed oil, 1 tbsp

- Chopped walnuts, .5 c

- Walnut milk, 2 c

- Shredded zucchini, 1 c

- Mashed burro banana, .25 c

- Date sugar, 2 tbsp

- Kamut flour or spelt, 2 c

What you'll do:

Place the date sugar and flour into a bowl. Whisk together.

Add in the mashed banana and walnut milk. Stir until combined. Remember to scrape the bowl to get all the dry mixture. Add in walnuts and zucchini. Stir well until combined.

Place the grapeseed oil onto a griddle and warm.

Pour .25 cup batter on the hot griddle. Leave it along until bubbles begin forming on to surface. Carefully turn over the pancake and cook another four minutes until cooked through.

Place the pancakes onto a serving plate and enjoy with some agave syrup.

Berry Sorbet

What you'll need:

- Water, 2 c

- Pureed strawberries, 2 c

- Spelt Flour, 1.5 tsp.

- Date sugar, .5 c

What you'll do:

Pour the water into a large pot and let the water begin to warm. Add the flour and date sugar and stir until dissolved. Allow this mixture to start boiling and continue to cook for around ten minutes. It should have started to thicken. Take off heat and set to the side to cool.

Once the syrup has cooled off, add in the strawberries, and stir well to combine.

Pour into a container that is freezer safe and put it into the freezer until frozen.

Take sorbet out of the freezer, cut into chunks, and put it either into a blender or a food processor. Hit the pulse button until the mixture is creamy.

Pour this into the same freezer-safe container and put it back into the freezer for four hours.

Quinoa Porridge

What you'll need:

- Zest of one lime

- Coconut milk, .5 c

- Cloves, .5 tsp.

- Ground ginger, 1.5 tsp.

- Springwater, 2 c

- Quinoa, 1 c

- Grated apple, 1

What you'll do:

Cook the quinoa according to the instructions on the package. When the quinoa has been cooked, drain well. Put it back into the pot and stir in spices.

Add coconut milk and stir well to combine.

Grate the apple now and stir well.

Divide equally into bowls and add the lime zest on top. Sprinkle with nuts and seeds of choice.

Apple Quinoa

What you'll need:

- Coconut oil, 1 tbsp
- Ginger
- Key lime .5
- Apple, 1
- Quinoa, .5 c
- Optional toppings
- Seeds
- Nuts
- Berries

What you'll do:

Fix the quinoa according to the instructions on the package. When you are getting close to the end of the cooking time, grate in the apple and cook for 30 seconds.

Zest the lime into the quinoa and squeeze the juice in. Stir in the coconut oil.

Divide evenly into bowls and sprinkle with some ginger.

You can add in some berries, nuts, and seeds right before you eat.

Kamut Porridge

What you'll need:

- Agave syrup, 4 tbsp

- Coconut oil, 1 tbsp

- Sea salt, .5 tsp.

- Coconut milk, 3.75 c

- Kamut berries, 1 c

- Optional toppings

- Berries

- Coconut chips

- Ground nutmeg

- Ground cloves

What you'll do:

You need to "crack" the Kamut berries. You can do this by placing the berries into a food processor and pulsing until you have 1.25 cups of Kamut.

Put the cracked Kamut in a pot with salt and coconut milk. Give it a good stir to combine everything. Allow this mixture to come to a full rolling boil and then turn the heat down until the mixture is simmering. Stir every now and then until the Kamut has thickened to your likeness. This normally takes about ten minutes.

Take off heat, stir in agave syrup and coconut oil.

Garnish with toppings of choice and enjoy.

Hot Kamut with Peaches, Walnuts, and Coconut

What you'll need:

- Toasted coconut, 4 tbsp

- Toasted and chopped walnuts, .5 c

- Chopped dried peaches, 8

- Coconut milk, 3 c

- Kamut cereal, 1 c

What you'll do:

Pour the coconut milk into a saucepan and allow it to warm up. When it begins simmering, add in the Kamut. Let this cook about 15 minutes, while stirring every now and then.

When done, divide evenly into bowls and top with the toasted coconut, walnuts, and peaches.

You could even go one more and add some fresh berries.

Kale Chickpea Mash

What you'll need:

- Sea salt, to taste
- Avocado oil, 2 tbsp
- Chickpeas, 1 15 oz can
- Kale, 1 bunch
- Onion, 1 small

What you'll do:

Dice the onion and place into a skillet of warmed avocado oil. Once onion is soft and slightly browned, add in the kale and stir well to combine. Cook until kale is softened.

Drain the chickpeas and add to kale. Cook about six minutes until chickpeas are warmed through. Pour into a blender and process until smooth.

Add sea salt to taste and stir well to combine.

Overnight "Oats"

What you'll need:

- Berry of choice, .5 c
- Walnut butter, .5 tbsp
- Burro banana, .5
- Ginger, .5 tsp.
- Coconut milk, .5 c
- Hemp seeds, .5 c

What you'll do:

Put the hemp seeds, salt, and coconut milk into a glass jar. Mix well.

Place the lid on the jar and put in the refrigerator to sit overnight.

The next morning, add the ginger, berries, and banana. Stir well and enjoy.

Blueberry Muffins

What you'll need:

- Grapeseed oil
- Sea salt, .5 tsp.
- Sea moss gel, .25 c
- Agave, .3 c
- Blueberries, .5 c
- Teff flour, .75 c
- Spelt flour, .75 c
- Coconut milk, 1 c

What you'll do:

Warm your oven to 365. Place paper liners into a muffin tin.

Place sea moss gel, sea salt, agave, flour, and milk in large bowl. Mix well to combine. Gently fold in blueberries.

Gently pour batter into paper liners. Place in oven and bake 30 minutes.

They are done when they have turned a nice golden color, and they spring back when you touch them.

Brazil Nut Cheese

What you'll need:

- Grapeseed oil, 2 tsp.

- Water, 1.5 c

- Hemp milk, 1.5 c

- Cayenne, .5 tsp.

- Onion powder, 1 tsp.

- Juice of .5 lime

- Sea salt, 2 tsp.

- Brazil nuts, 1 lb.

- Onion powder, 1 tsp.

What you'll do:

You will need to start by soaking the Brazil nuts in some water. You just put the nuts into a bowl and make sure the water covers them. Soak no less than two hours or overnight. Overnight would be best.

Now you need to put everything except water into a food processor or blender.

Add just .5 cups water and blend for two minutes

Continue adding .5 cup water and blending until you have the consistency you want.

Scrape into an airtight container and enjoy.

Baked Stuffed Pears

What you'll need:

- Agave syrup, 4 tbsp

- Cloves, .25 tsp.

- Chopped walnuts, 4 tbsp

- Currants, 1 c

- Pears, 4

What you'll do:

Make sure your oven has been warmed to 375.

Slice the pears in two lengthwise and remove the core. To get the pear to lay flat, you can slice a small piece off the back side.

Place the agave syrup, currants, walnuts, and cloves in a small bowl and mix well. Set this to the side to be used later.

Put the pears on a cookie sheet that has parchment paper on it. Make sure the cored sides are facing up. Sprinkle each pear half with about .5 tablespoon of the chopped walnut mixture.

Place into the oven and cook for 25 to 30 minutes. Pears should be tender.

Butternut Squash Pie

What you'll need:

- For the Crust
- Cold water
- Agave, splash
- Sea salt, pinch
- Grapeseed oil, .5 c
- Coconut flour, .5 c
- Spelt Flour, 1 c
- For the Filling
- Butternut squash, peeled, chopped
- Water
- Allspice, to taste
- Agave syrup, to taste
- Hemp milk, 1 c
- Sea moss, 4 tbsp

What you'll do:

You will need to warm your oven to 350.

For the Crust

Place the grapeseed oil and water into the refrigerator to get it cold. This will take about one hour.

Place all ingredients into a large bowl. Now you need to add in the cold water a little bit in small amounts until a dough forms. Place this onto a surface that has been sprinkled with some coconut flour. Knead for a few minutes and roll the dough as thin as you can get it. Carefully pick it up and place it inside a pie plate.

Place the butternut squash into a Dutch oven and pour in enough water to cover. Bring this to a full rolling boil. Let this cook until the squash has become soft.

Completely drain and place into bowl. Using a potato masher, mash the squash. Add in some allspice and agave to taste. Add in the sea moss and hemp milk. Using a hand mixer, blend well. Pour into the pie crust.

Place into the oven and bake for about one hour.

Cheesecake

What you need

Cheesecake:

- Sea salt, .25 tsp.

- Sea moss gel, 1 tbsp

- Lime juice, 2 tbsp

- Dates, 5 to 6

- Agave, .25 c

- Hemp or walnut milk, 1.5 c

- Brazil nuts, 2 c

- Crust:

- Sea salt, .25 tsp.

- Agave, .25 c

- Coconut flakes, 1.5 c

- Dates, 1.5 c

Topping:

- Blackberries

- Blueberries

- Sliced raspberries

- Sliced strawberry

- Sliced mango

What you'll do:

Add all of the crust ingredients into your food processor and blend it for about 20 seconds.

Spread your crust out into a springform pan that has been covered with parchment.

Place the mango slices along the side of the pan and then place it in the freezer as you prepare everything else.

Add everything for the cheesecake to your blender and mix it together until it creates a smooth mixture.

Remove the springform pan from the freezer and pour the filling in. Wrap in foil and let it sit for three to four hours.

Carefully remove from the pan, and then place the rest of the toppings over the top. All of the leftovers should be kept in the freezer.

Blackberry Jam

What you'll need:

- Sea moss gel, .75 c

- Key lime juice, 1 tbsp

- Agave nectar, 3 tbsp

- Blackberries, 3 – six-ounce packages

What you'll do:

Rinse the blackberries under cold water.

Place them in a pot and place over medium heat. Stir until the blackberries begin the release their juices.

When the blackberries begin to breakdown, take an immersion blender, and process any large pieces of blackberries. If immersion isn't an option, you can just mash them with a potato masher or put in a blender to process them.

Now, add in the sea moss gel, key lime juice, and agave nectar. Stir until the jam begins to thicken.

Take off heat and let cool for 15 minutes.

You can use this in any way you would like.

If you don't use all of this at one time, place in a glass jar with a lid. Can be stored in the refrigerator for up to one week. This can also be stored in the freezer for up to two months.

Blackberry Bars

What you'll need:

- Blackberry jam, 1 c (recipe above)
- Sea salt, .25 tsp.
- Spelt Flour, 1 c
- Quinoa flakes, 2 c
- Agave nectar, .25 c
- Grapeseed oil, .5 c
- Burro bananas, 3

What you'll do:

You need to warm your oven to 350.

Using a potato masher or fork, mash the bananas in a large bowl.

Add in the agave nectar and grapeseed oil and stir well to combine.

Add the spelt flour and quinoa flakes to this mixture. Mix together until it forms a dough that is sticky.

Place a piece of parchment paper into a square baking dish. Press the dough into the pan evenly.

Spread the blackberry jam evenly on top of the dough.

Crumble the remaining dough in clumps on top of jam.

Place in preheated oven for 20 minutes. When it is done, take out of oven and let cool for 15 minutes before you cut them.

You can store these in the fridge for up to six days or freeze for three months.

Pumpkin Pie

What you'll need:

- For Crust
- Cloves, 1 tsp.
- Coconut flakes, 1 c
- Dates, 1 c
- Raw walnuts, 1 c
- For Filling
- Sea salt, .25 tsp.
- Nutmeg, .5 tsp.
- Cloves, .5 tsp.
- Dates, 6
- Pumpkin puree, 1.25 c
- Walnuts, 1 c

What you'll do:

For Crust:

Place the walnuts, dates, coconut flakes, and cloves into a food processor. Process until you begin to see the oils coming out, and it begins to stick together. Pour this mixture into a nine-inch pie pan or tart mold. Press against the bottom and sides.

For Filling:

Place all the filling ingredients into a blender. Turn on the blender until all the ingredients have come together in a smooth liquid. Pour this mixture in the pie crust. If you would like, you can sprinkle with some nutmeg. Put in the refrigerator to mold and get cold.

Blueberry Pancakes

What you'll need:

- Grapeseed oil
- Hemp seeds, 2 tbsp
- Bromide powder or sea moss, .25 tsp.
- Blueberries, .5 c
- Agave, .5 c
- Grapeseed oil, 2 tbsp
- Springwater, .5 c
- Hemp milk, 1 c
- Spelt Flour, 2 c

What you'll do:

Combine the grapeseed oil, agave, sea moss, hemp seeds, and spelt flour together.

Stir in a cup of hemp milk, and stir in enough spring water until it reaches the consistency you like.

Fold in the blueberries.

Heat up your skillet and coat it with some grapeseed oil.

Add some of the batter to your skillet and cook the pancakes for three to five minutes on both sides. Enjoy.

Banana Cream Pie

What you'll need:

Filling:

- Sea salt, pinch
- Agave, 3 to 4 tbsp
- Hemp milk, 1 c
- Creamed coconut, 7 oz
- Baby bananas, 6 to 8

Crust:

- Sea salt, .25 tsp.
- Agave, .25 c
- Unsweetened coconut flakes, 1.5 c
- Pitted dates, 1.5 c

What you'll do:

Add the crust ingredients to your food processor and mix it until it creates a ball.

Add some parchment paper to your springform pan. Spread your crust evenly across the pan.

Thinly slice the bananas and lay them along the inside of the pan. Place it in the freezer.

Place the filling mixture into a bowl and use an electric mixer to mix it all together.

Pour the filling into the pan. Shake the pan to even out the filling. Cover the pan with the foil and place it back in the freezer for three to four hours.

Top the cake with coconut and enjoy.

Date Balls

What you'll need:

- Sea salt, .5 tsp.

- Agave nectar, .25 c

- Sesame seeds, .5 c

- Walnuts or brazil nuts, .5 c

- Unsweetened coconut flakes or coconut meat, 1 c

- Pitted dates, 1 c

What you'll do:

This is a very easy recipe to put together. All you need to do is add everything, minus the sesame seeds, to your food processor. Press the pulse button five times and then turn it on to blend for 20 seconds or until it is all well blended.

This next step might be easier if you wet your hands slightly. Take a spoonful of the date mixture out and roll it between your palms until it becomes a ball. After you roll a ball, roll it into some sesame seeds. Continue until you have used all of the date mixture. Make sure that you keep the date balls stored in an airtight container. Enjoy.

Chapter 3: Smoothies

Orange Creamsicle

What you'll need:

- Bromide Plus Powder, .5 tsp.

- Date sugar, to taste

- Coconut water, 1 c

- Burro banana, .5

- Seville oranges, 3 peeled

What you'll do:

Place the oranges, banana, coconut water, date sugar, and bromide plus powder into a blender. Turn the blender on until it forms a creamy drink.

Green Detox

What you'll need:

- Soft jelly coconut water, .5 c

- Blueberries, .25 c

- Ginger tea, .5 c

- Key lime juice, 2 to 3 tbsp

- Romaine lettuce, 1 c

- Burro banana, .5

What you'll do:

Fix the tea according to directions on the package. Set to the side and allow to cool.

Once the tea is cool, you will need to put everything into a blender. Turn the blender on and leave it until it turns into a creamy drink.

Iron Power

What you'll need:

- Bromide Plus Powder, 1 tsp.

- Date sugar, 1 tbsp

- Amaranth greens, 2 handfuls

- Hemp seed milk, 1 c homemade

- Cooked quinoa, .5 c

- Fig, 1

- Raisins or currants, 1 tbsp

- Large red apple, .5

What you'll do:

Place the apple, raisins, fig, quinoa, milk, greens, sugar, and bromide plus powder into your blender. Turn the blender on and let run until a creamy drink has been made.

Sweet Sunrise

What you'll need:

- Water, 1 c

- Mango, 1 c

- Burro banana, .5

- Seville orange, 1

- Raspberries, 1 c

What you'll do:

Place the raspberries, orange, banana, mango, and water into your blender. Turn the blender on and let run until it forms a creamy drink.

Coconut Lime

What you'll need:

- Springwater, .5 c
- Ice, 1 c
- Key limes, 2 peeled
- Fresh coconut meat, 1 c
- Avocado, 1
- Kale, handful
- Cucumber, .5 c

What you'll do:

Place all the above ingredients into a blender and process until creamy and smooth.

Super Shake

What you'll need:

- Agave syrup, .25 tsp.
- Coconut oil, 1 tsp.
- Juice of one key lime
- Hemp seeds, 1 tbsp
- Fresh parsley, 1 tbsp
- Coconut water, .5 c
- Avocado, 1
- Fresh ginger, 1 tbsp
- Kale leaves, 2 stalks removed
- Cucumber, .5 c

What you'll do:

Put all of the above ingredients in your blender. Turn on the blender and let it work until it forms a creamy drink. Try to drink it within 15 minutes of making it to get the best benefits.

Alkaline Smoothie

What you'll need:

- Ice, 1 c
- Hemp seeds, 1 tsp.
- Dandelion greens, handful
- Burro banana, .5
- Frozen strawberries, 5
- Cubed watermelon, 1 c
- Coconut milk, 1 c

What you'll do:

Carefully cut your watermelon in half and cut it into cubes. Remove seeds and place them in a glass container. Put in the fridge to get cold.

Wash the strawberries and cut the caps off. Place in a freezer-safe container and freeze until needed.

Wash the kale. Remove stalks and chop into bite-size pieces.

In order not to have a brown smoothie, put the greens and the banana together, half the milk, half the ice, and the hemp seeds. Process until creamy and smooth. Pour this into a glass.

Now add the rest of the ice, milk, strawberries, and watermelon. Process until creamy and smooth. Pour this on top of the other smoothie.

Apple Banana

What you'll need:

- Ice, 1 c
- Hemp seeds, 1 tsp.
- Coconut milk, 1 c
- Nutmeg, 1 tsp.
- Burro banana, 1
- Apple, 1

What you'll do:

Peel and core the apple and put it in a blender.

Roughly chop the banana and put it in the blender.

Add all the other ingredients into the blender. Turn the blender on and let it run until you have a creamy drink.

Mango Strawberry

What you'll need:

- Frozen mango, 1 c
- Frozen burro banana, 1
- Strawberries, 5
- Water, .25 c
- Juice of one Seville orange, .75 c

What you'll do:

Wash the strawberries and cut off the caps.

Peel the mango and place it in the freezer to freeze until ready to use.

Roughly chop the banana and put it in the freezer until ready to use.

Pour the orange juice and water into the blender.

Add mango, banana, and strawberries. You can add a teaspoon of hemp seeds now if you would like.

Process until creamy and smooth.

Strawberry Banana Quinoa

What you'll need:

- Agave syrup, 1 tsp.

- Quinoa, .75 c

- Burro banana, 1 large

- Strawberries, 10

- Coconut milk, 1 c

What you'll do:

Place the quinoa into a bowl and cover with water. Let sit for two hours. Drain well.

Roughly chop the banana and put it in the freezer until ready to use.

Wash the strawberries and cut off the caps.

Put the coconut milk, strawberries, banana, quinoa, and syrup into your blender. Turn the blender on and let it run until you have a creamy drink.

You can use more or fewer strawberries according to your taste. It gets pinker when you use more strawberries.

Glowing Green Smoothie

What you'll need:

- Ice cubes, 2 c

- Sea salt, pinch

- Agave syrup, to taste

- Limes, halved and peeled, 2 medium

- Zest of one key lime

- English cucumber, .5

- Avocado, pitted and peeled

- Amaranth greens, 2 c

- Coconut water, .75 c

What you'll do:

Zest the key lime. Remove the peel. Set segments to the side.

Take the English cucumber and peel it, cut it into chunks.

Slice the avocado in two lengthwise and carefully take the pit out and peel.

Wash the greens and put them in the blender.

Put all the other ingredients into your blender. Turn the blender on and let it run until you have a creamy drink.

Alkaline Boosting Smoothie

What you'll need:

- Ice cubes, 1 c

- Kale, handful

- Seville orange, 1

- Burro banana, .5

- Cucumber, .25

- Coconut milk, .25 c

What you'll do:

Peel the cucumber and cut one-fourth of it off. Place in the blender.

Wash the kale and cut into bite-size pieces.

Peel the orange and set the segments to the side.

When you are ready to make the smoothie, make sure all of your ingredients are in your blender. Turn the blender on and let it run until you have a creamy drink.

Aloha Breakfast Smoothie

What you'll need:

- Ice, 1 c
- Coconut water, .5 c
- Orange, peeled
- Smashed ginger root, 1 inch
- Chopped cucumber, .5
- Kale, 2 handfuls
- Avocado, 1

What you'll do:

Wash the kale and chop it into bite-size pieces. Place in blender.

Slice the avocado open and carefully take out the pit. Scoop out the flesh from the peel. Put in the blender with the kale.

Peel the orange and place the segments into the blender.

Smash the ginger root and chop small. Place into the blender.

Peel and seed the cucumber. Chop in bite-size pieces and put in the blender with the rest of the other ingredients.

Turn your blender on and let it run until you have a creamy drink.

Green Detox Smoothie

What you'll need:

- Agave syrup, to taste
- Ice, handful
- Coconut water, 1 c
- Parsley, handful
- Cucumber, .5
- Ginger root, 1 inch
- Key lime, 5 peeled
- Turnip greens, handful

What you'll do:

Wash the turnip greens and place them in the blender.

Cut one inch off of a ginger root and smash it, then chop into small pieces. Place into the blender

Peel the key lime and place the segments into the blender.

Wash the parsley and place into the blender.

Add all the other ingredients into your blender. Turn the blender on and let it run until you have a creamy drink.

Avocado Detox

What you'll need:

- Coconut butter, 1 tbsp
- Ginger root, 1 inch
- Amaranth greens, large handful
- Cucumber, 1
- Avocado, 1
- Coconut water, 1 c

What you'll do:

Peel and chop the cucumber and put it in the blender.

Cut the avocado lengthwise and twist apart. Carefully remove the pit and scoop out the flesh into the blender.

Wash the amaranth greens and roughly tear. Put them in the blender.

Cut one inch off of a ginger root and cut into small pieces.

Place the other ingredients into your blender. Turn the blender on and let it run until you have a creamy drink.

Pumpkin Spice Smoothie

What you'll need:

- Hemp seeds, 1 tbsp
- Date, 1
- Nutmeg, .25 tsp.
- Ground ginger, .25 tsp.
- Cloves, .25 tsp.
- Frozen banana, 1
- Pumpkin, 1 c
- Coconut milk, 2 c
- Kale, 2 c

What you'll do:

Wash the kale and chop it into bite-size pieces, place it into the blender. Add the coconut milk and process until smooth.

If you are using a fresh pumpkin, carefully cut open the pumpkin and scoop out the seeds. Peel the pumpkin and chop into bite-size pieces. You can freeze the rest of the pumpkin to be used at a later date.

Place the pumpkin in the blender along with the frozen banana, cloves, ginger, nutmeg, and date. Process until creamy and smooth.

Add the hemp seeds last and pulse a few times to combine.

Summer Berry

What you'll need:

- Coconut water, 1 c
- Nutmeg, 1 tsp.
- Juice of one key lime
- Hemp seeds, 1 tbsp
- Frozen banana, .5
- Coconut oil, 1 tbsp
- Mixed berries, .5 c
- Turnip greens, large handful

What you'll do:

Wash the turnip greens and place them in the blender.

Wash the berries and place them in the blender.

Add the frozen banana, key lime juice, nutmeg, coconut oil, coconut water, and hemp seeds to the blender. Process all until creamy and smooth.

Liquid Fat-Burning Smoothie

What you'll need:

- Ice, handful
- Hemp seeds, 1 tbsp
- Raw walnut butter, 1 tbsp
- Frozen banana, 1
- Avocado, 1
- Coconut milk, 1 c

What you'll do:

Cut the avocado lengthwise and twist apart. Carefully remove the pit and scoop out the flesh. Place the flesh into the blender.

Add the remaining ingredients to the blender and process until creamy and smooth.

Hearty Power Smoothie

What you'll need:

- Ground ginger, .5 tsp.

- Coconut oil, 1 tbsp

- Kamut, .33 c

- Frozen banana, 1

- Green apple, 1

- Coconut milk, 2 c

- Turnip greens, 2 c

What you'll do:

Wash the turnip greens and place them in the blender.

Peel and core the apple, place it into the blender.

Add all the other ingredients into your blender. Turn the blender on and let it run until you have a creamy drink.

Berry Good Kale Smoothie

What you'll need:

- Raw tahini butter, 2 tbsp
- Cloves, .5 tsp.
- Coconut milk, 2 c
- Coconut oil, 1 tbsp
- Frozen banana, 1
- Frozen mixed berries, 1 c
- Kale, 2 c

What you'll do:

Wash the kale and chop it into bite-size pieces. Place it into the blender.

Put all the remaining ingredients in your blender. Turn the blender on and let it run until you have a creamy drink.

Tahini Butter Crunch Smoothie

What you'll need:

- Hemp seeds, 1 tbsp
- Coconut milk, 2 c
- Raw tahini butter, 4 tbsp
- Frozen banana, 1
- Frozen mixed berries, 1 c
- Turnip greens, 2 c

What you'll do:

Wash the turnip greens and place them into the blender.

Add the remaining ingredients to the blender and process until creamy and smooth.

Raspberry Lime Smoothie

What you'll need:

- Hemp seeds, 1 tbsp

- Coconut milk, 1 c

- Juice of one key lime

- Raspberries, 1 c

- Kale, handful

- Ice, 1 c

What you'll do:

Wash the kale and chop into bite-size pieces. Place into the blender.

Wash the raspberries and place them into the blender with the kale.

Add all the other ingredients in your blender. Turn the blender on and let it run until you have a creamy drink.

"Cinnamon" Bun Smoothie

What you'll need:

- Hemp seeds, 1 tbsp

- Cloves, .75 tsp.

- Pitted date, 1

- Raw tahini butter, 2 tbsp

- Frozen banana, 1

- Kale, large handful

- Coconut milk, 1 c

What you'll do:

Wash the kale and place it in the blender.

Place all the other ingredients into your blender. Turn the blender on and let it run until you have a creamy drink.

Summer Citrus Smoothie

What you'll need:

- Frozen banana, 1
- Juice of one key lime
- Romaine lettuce heart, .5
- Cucumber, .5
- Kale, handful
- Orange, 1
- Coconut water, .5 c

What you'll do:

Wash the Romaine lettuce. Chop into bite-size pieces and place in the blender.

Peel the orange and tear into segments. Place the segments into the blender with the lettuce.

Juice the lime and place it into the blender with the lettuce and orange.

Peel the cucumber. Chop into bite-size pieces and place in the blender with the orange, lettuce, and lime juice.

Add any ingredient you haven't used yet into your blender. Turn the blender on and let it run until you have a creamy drink.

Lean, Green Protein Smoothie

What you'll need:

- Coconut flakes, 1 tbsp
- Raw tahini butter, 1 tbsp
- Kale, handful
- Hemp seeds, 1 tbsp
- Amaranth greens, handful
- Frozen butter, 1
- Coconut water, .75 c
- Coconut milk, .5 c

What you'll do:

Wash the kale and chop into bite-size pieces. Place into the blender.

Wash the amaranth greens and chop into bite-size pieces. Place this with the kale in your blender.

Add all the ingredients that you haven't used into your blender. Turn the blender on and let it run until you have a creamy drink.

Spring Ahead Smoothie

What you'll need:

- Coconut milk, 1 c
- Hemp seeds, 1 tbsp
- Frozen banana, 1
- Coconut oil, 1 tbsp
- Blueberries, .5 c
- Turnip greens, 2 c

What you'll do:

Wash the turnip greens and chop into bite-size pieces. Place into the blender.

Wash the blueberries and place them in the blender with the turnip greens.

Add the remaining ingredients to the blender and process until creamy and smooth.

Blueberry Morning Blast

What you'll need:

- Coconut milk, 1 c
- Coconut oil, 1 tbsp
- Hemp seed powder, 3 tbsp
- Raw tahini butter, 1 tbsp
- Blueberries, .5 c
- Kale, large handful

What you'll do:

Wash the kale and chop into bite-size pieces. Place into a blender.

Wash the blueberries and put them into the blender.

Add the remaining ingredients to the blender and process until creamy and smooth.

Blackberry Smoothie

What you'll need:

- Raw walnut butter, 1 tbsp

- Coconut oil, 2 tbsp

- Juice of one key lime

- Kale, large handful

- Frozen strawberries, .5 c

- Frozen blackberries, 1 c

- Coconut milk, 1.5 c

What you'll do:

Wash the kale and chop into bite-size pieces. Place into a blender

Add coconut milk and process until smooth.

Add any ingredient that you haven't used yet into your blender. Turn the blender on and let it run until you have a creamy drink.

Winter Green Smoothie

What you'll need:

- Hemp seeds, 1 tbsp
- Pear, 1
- Frozen banana, .5
- Coconut oil, 1 tbsp
- Kale, handful
- Coconut water, 1 c
- Nutmeg, pinch

What you'll do:

Wash the kale and chop into bite-size pieces. Place into a blender.

Wash the pear. Peel and core the pear and chop into bite-size pieces. Place into the blender.

Add any ingredient to the blender that you haven't used yet. Turn the blender on and let it run until you have a creamy drink.

Coco Loco Smoothie

What you'll need:

- Frozen banana, 1
- Coconut oil, 1 tbsp
- Coconut water, 1 c
- Coconut meat, 4 oz
- Ice, 1 c

What you'll do:

Put the ice, coconut meat, coconut water, coconut oil, and banana in your blender. Turn your blender on and let it run until you have a creamy drink.

Glorious Breakfast Smoothie

What you'll need:

- Coconut water, .5 c
- Plum, 1
- Cucumber, .5
- Turnip greens, handful
- Kale, .5 bunch

What you'll do:

Wash the kale and chop into bite-size pieces. Place into a blender.

Peel the cucumber and chop into bite-size pieces. Put into the blender with the kale.

Wash the turnip greens and chop into bite-size pieces. Place in the blender with the cucumber and kale.

Slice the plum around the seam and pry it apart. Remove the pit and discard. Slice the plum and put it into the blender with the greens.

Add the coconut water and process until creamy and smooth.

Berry Peach Smoothie

What you'll need:

- Frozen cherries, .5 c
- Coconut water, 1 c
- Sea moss gel, 1 tbsp
- Frozen peaches, .5 c
- Agave, 1 tbsp
- Frozen strawberries, .5 c
- Hemp seeds, 1 tbsp
- Frozen blueberries, .5 c

What you'll do:

Begin by placing all of the above ingredients into your blender and mix together until it creates a smooth drink. If you find that it is too thick, you can add a bit more coconut water.

Apple Pie

What you'll need:

- Bromide Plus Powder, 1 tsp.

- Date sugar, 1 tbsp

- Ginger tea, 1 c

- Walnuts, handful

- Figs, 2

- Large apple, .5

What you'll do:

Fix the ginger tea according to the package directions. Set it to the side and let it cool down.

Once cooled, add to a blender along with all the rest of the above ingredients. Process until creamy and smooth.

Veggie-Ful

What you'll need:

- Date sugar, to taste
- Water, .5 c
- Romaine lettuce, handful
- Watercress, handful
- Cucumber, peeled and seeded, .5
- Avocado, .25
- Pear, seeded, cored, 1

What you'll do:

Place the pear, avocado, cucumber, watercress, lettuce, water, and sugar into your blender. Turn the blender on and let it run until you have a creamy drink.

Energizing

What you'll need:

- Bromide Plus Powder, 1 tsp.

- Date sugar, 1 tbsp

- Cooked amaranth or quinoa, .5 c

- Hemp milk, 1 c

- Papaya, 1 c

What you'll do:

Place the bromide powder, sugar, cooked quinoa, milk, and papaya into your blender. Turn the blender on and let it run until you have a drink that is creamy.

Tropical Breeze

What you'll need:

- Amaranth greens, handful

- Soft jelly coconut water, 1 c

- Burro banana, .5

- Watermelon, .5 c

- Cantaloupe, .5 c

- Mango, .5

What you'll do:

Place the greens, water, banana, watermelon, cantaloupe, and mango into your blender. Turn on the blender and let it run until you have a creamy drink.

Super Hydrating

What you'll need:

- Date sugar, 1 tbsp

- Soft jelly coconut water, 1 c

- Watermelon chunks, 1 c

- Strawberries, 1 c

What you'll do:

Place the strawberries, watermelon, water, and sugar into your blender. Turn on your blender and let it run until you have a creamy drink.

Sea Moss Green

What you'll need:

- Mixed greens, 2 c

- Burro banana, 1

- Sea moss, 2 tbsp

What you'll do:

Wash the greens and place in a blender. Place all the other ingredients into your blender. Turn the blender on and let it run until you have a creamy drink.

Mango Banana

What you'll need:

- Water, 1 c

- Greens, 2 c

- Burro banana, .5

- Mango, 1

What you'll do:

Wash the greens and place them into a blender. Peel the mango and cut the fruit off the core. Place into the blender with the greens. Add all the other ingredients to your blender. Turn the blender on and let it run until you have a creamy drink.

Kale Berry Delight

What you'll need:

- Coconut milk, 1 c

- Kale, 2 c

- Apple, 1 large

- Mixed berries, 1 c

What you'll do:

Wash the kale and tear it into pieces, place into a blender. Peel and core the apple, place it into the blender with the kale. Add any ingredient you haven't used yet into your blender. Turn the blender on and let it run until you have a creamy drink.

Banana Coconut

What you'll need:

- Kale, 2 c
- Coconut water, 1 c
- Pear, 1
- Burro banana, 1

What you'll do:

Wash and chop the kale, place into a blender.

Peel and core the pear and chop into pieces. Put it into the blender with the kale.

Add any other ingredient you have used yet into your blender. Turn the blender on and let it run until you have a creamy drink.

Apple Juice Mix

What you'll need:

- Avocado, .5

- Apple, 1

- Kale, 2 c

- Apple juice, 1.5 c

What you'll do:

Wash the kale. Stem and tear into pieces. Place into a blender.

Peel and core the apple. Chop into pieces. Put it into the blender with the kale.

Add any ingredient you haven't used yet to your blender. Turn the blender on and let it run until you have a creamy drink.

Banana Flax

What you'll need:

- Water, 1 c
- Flax seeds, 1 tbsp
- Frozen banana, 1
- Blueberries, .5 c
- Greens, 2 c

What you'll do:

Wash the greens and blueberries and place them into a blender.

Add any ingredient that you haven't used yet into your blender. Turn the blender on and let it run until you have a creamy drink.

Fresh Greens

What you'll need:

- Date, 1
- Coconut water, 1 c
- Cucumber, .5
- Fresh ginger, 1 inch
- Key lime, .5
- Greens, handful

What you'll do:

Wash the greens and place them into a blender. Peel the cucumber and cut into pieces. Place into the blender with the greens. Peel the ginger using a spoon and slice into thin slices before putting it in the blender. If you put the whole inch of ginger into the blender, it will make your drink very fibrous. Basically, it will feel like you are trying to drink hair. I know... gross.

Back to the instructions.

Put any ingredient you haven't used yet into your blender. Turn the blender on and let it run until you have a creamy drink.

Banana Berry Kale

What you'll need:

- Ice, 1 c
- Kale, 1 c
- Strawberries, frozen or fresh, 1 c
- Burro banana, 1

What you'll do:

Wash the kale and chop it. Place it into the blender.

Wash and cap the strawberries and place them into the blender with the kale.

Add any other ingredient you haven't used into your blender. Turn the blender on and let it run until you have a creamy drink.

Apple Berries

What you'll need:

- Water, 1 c
- Greens, 2 c
- Apple, 1 large
- Mixed berries, 1 c

What you'll do:

Wash the greens and place them into the blender.

Peel and core the apple and chop into pieces. Add to the greens in the blender.

Place any ingredient you haven't used yet into your blender. Turn the blender on and let it run until you have a creamy drink.

Raspberry Greens

What you'll need:

- Sea moss, 1 tbsp
- Coconut milk, 1 c
- Key lime juice, 2 tbsp
- Frozen raspberries, 1 c
- Leafy greens, handful

What you'll do:

Wash the greens and place them into a blender.

Add the other ingredients to your blender. Turn on the blender and let it run until you have a creamy drink.

Berry Sea Moss

What you'll need:

- Coconut water, 1 c
- Sea moss, 1 tbsp
- Juice of one key lime
- Frozen burro banana, .5
- Mixed berries, .5 c
- Greens, large handful

What you'll do:

Wash the greens and place them into the blender.

Put any ingredient you haven't used yet into your blender. Turn your blender on and let it run until you have a creamy drink.

Sea Moss Apple Pie Smoothie

What you'll need:

- Ice cubes, 2 c
- Clove powder, dash
- Fresh ginger, 1 tbsp
- Sea moss gel, heaping tbsp
- Fresh apple juice, 2 c

What you'll do:

Place everything from above into your blender and mix until blended. Enjoy.

Spicy Green Smoothie

What you'll need:

- Sea moss gel, 1 tbsp

- Lime juice, .25 c

- Spring water, 2 c

- Thumb of ginger

- Cucumber, 1 c

- Apple

- Kale, 2 handfuls

What you'll do:

Add everything to your blender and mix for a couple of minutes, or until it is blended to your liking. Enjoy.

Crisp Green Smoothie

What you'll need:

- Sea moss gel, 1 tbsp
- Lime juice, .25 c
- Springwater, 2 c
- Thumb of ginger
- Dates, 6
- Honeydew, .25
- Cucumber, 1 c
- Pear
- Bunch of arugulas
- Bunch of callaloo

What you'll do:

Add everything to your blender and mix for a couple of minutes, or until it reaches your desired consistency. Enjoy.

Fruity Green Smoothie

What you'll need:

- Burdock root powder, 1 tbsp

- Lime juice, .25 c

- Springwater, 2 c

- Thumb of ginger

- Dates, 6

- Baby bananas, 3

- Blueberries, .5 c

- Handful of watercress

- Bunch of dandelion greens

What you'll do:

Add all of the ingredients to a blender and mix for a couple of minutes, or until it reaches your desired consistency. Enjoy.

Triple Berry Smoothie

What you'll need:

- Agave
- Burro banana
- Water, 1 c
- Blueberries, .5 c
- Raspberries, .5 c
- Strawberries, .5 c

What you'll do:

Begin by washing the fruit. Peel and dice the banana. Add the fruit to the blender. Begin blending and slowly add the water in until it reaches the consistency you like. Blend in some agave to taste.

Toxin Flush Smoothie

What you'll need:

- A key lime

- A cucumber

- Cubed, seeded watermelon, 1 c

What you'll do:

Wash and dice the cucumber. Add the watermelon and cucumber to the blender and mix until combined. You shouldn't need to add extra water since both the watermelon and cucumber are mainly water.

Slice the lime in half and squeeze the juice into your smoothie. Enjoy.

Detoxifying Smoothie

What you'll need:

- A key lime

- A quarter of an avocado

- Amaranth greens, 2 c

- Cored apples, 2

- Water, 2 c

What you'll do:

Begin by cleaning the apples and amaranth greens. If your blender is a high speed one, you should peel the apples first. Add the apples, greens, and avocado to a blender. Mix everything together in the blender and slowly add the water into the mixture until it reaches your desired consistency. Juice the lime into your smoothie and mix together.

Detox Berry Smoothie

What you'll need:

- A quarter of an avocado

- Water

- Hemp seeds, 1 tbsp

- Fresh lettuce, 2 c

- Mixture of your favorite berries, 1 c

- Seville orange

- Burro banana

What you'll do:

Wash your berries. Peel the orange and banana. Segment the orange out and slice the banana. Add the berries, orange, banana, lettuce, and avocado to the blender. Start mixing them all together, and slowly add in the water until it reaches the consistency you like. Mix in the hemp seeds and enjoy.

Blissful Smoothie

What you'll need:

- Water, 1 c
- Cooked quinoa, .25 c
- Blueberries, 1 oz
- A quarter of an avocado
- Chopped pear

What you'll do:

You first need to start by cooking your quinoa and allowing it to cool completely. This is a good recipe to do the morning after you have had quinoa for dinner.

Then wash your fruit and chop up the pear. Add the quinoa, blueberries, avocado, and pear to your blender. Being mixing everything together and slowly add in the water until it reaches your desired consistency. Enjoy.

Apple Blueberry Smoothie

What you'll need:

- Bromide plus powder, .5 tbsp
- A date
- Sesame seeds, 1 tbsp
- Soft-jelly coconut water, 2 c
- Hemp seeds, 1 tbsp
- Callaloo, .5 c
- A half of an apple
- Blueberries, .5 c

What you'll do:

Begin by washing and dicing your apple. You can also peel the apple if your blender doesn't mix things up perfectly. Wash the blueberries, and then add the fruit to your blender and along with all of the other ingredients. Mix everything together and enjoy.

Green Veggie Berry Smoothie

What you'll need:

- Spring water, 1 c
- Handful of your favorite approved berries
- Burro banana
- Favorite approved greens, 2 c

What you'll do:

Begin by washing your berries and greens. Peel and slice your banana and then add all of the fruits and veggies into your blender. Begin to blend everything together and slowly add in the water until the smoothie reaches the consistency that you like. Enjoy.

Banana "Ice Cream" Smoothie

What you'll need:

- Ginger, .5 tsp.

- Springwater, 1 c

- Approved nut butter, 1 tbsp

- A handful of raisins

- Frozen, sliced burro bananas, 2

What you'll do:

Begin by placing the raisins into a bowl of water and allow them to soak for at least two hours. This will help the texture of smoothie so that it doesn't become grainy.

Once the raisins have soaked long enough, add them along with the bananas, nut butter, and ginger to your blender. Begin blending everything together and slowly add in the spring water until it reaches your desired consistency. Enjoy.

Prickly Pear Smoothie

What you'll need:

- Ginger, .5 tsp.

- Springwater, .5 c

- Burro bananas, 2

- Prickly pear juice, 1 c*

What you'll do:

First off, we will make the prickly pear juice.

You will take two prickly pears, make sure they are cleaned, and add them to your blender along with a cup of water. Mix everything together and then strain the juice through some cheesecloth. If you have a juicer, you can also run the prickly pears through it. The juicing method won't give you as much liquid, so your smoothie will end up being thicker.

Next, slice your bananas and them along with the prickly pear juice and ginger to your blender. Begin mixing them together and slowly add in the spring water until it reaches your desired consistency. Enjoy.

"Pretty in Pink" Smoothie

What you'll need:

- Burro banana

- Small apple

- A handful of your favorite berries, frozen

What you'll do:

First, you will want to make sure you wash your fruit before you place them in the freezer to freeze. Then peel and chop your apple and slice the banana. Add all of the fruit to your blender and mix everything together. If the smoothie is too thick for you, you can blend in some spring water to thin it out some. Enjoy.

Chapter 4: Herbal Recipes

Herbs are a big part of Dr. Sebi's diet, but there are only certain ones that you can consume. Each plays a big part in the diet. The herbs we will talk about are most commonly used in Dr. Sebi's supplements, but you will see in the recipes, there are many other herbs you can use as well. Let's take a look at the herbs before we get into the recipes.

- **Burdock Root**: This herb helps to increase your circulation and will detoxify the epidermis, which makes it great for treating a large number of skin conditions, like acne, psoriasis, abscesses, eczema, and carbuncles. It is also believed to be great at fighting off fungi and bacteria. This plant is a powerhouse of antioxidants and can help to protect your cells from damage. Due to all of its antioxidant power, herbalists like to use burdock root to prevent and treat many different health problems.

- **Bladderwrack**: This is rich in iodine, and helps to boost your metabolism because it stimulates your thyroid. It also helps to fight off obesity and cellulite. You can either consume it or use it externally to help with inflammation and joint pain.

- **Black Cumin**: This is one of the best anti-inflammatory herbs.

- **Blessed Thistle**: This herb has the ability to cure several different ailments. It is sometimes referred to as St. Benedict's Thistle or Holy Thistle. Many herbalists do refer to this as a gift from God, especially for women. Blessed thistle can help in working through many female related problems. It can help to increase breast milk supply, and it can also fix a hormonal imbalance. It also holds astringent compounds that can help to calm inflamed tissues and dilate peripheral blood vessels.

186

- **Blue Vervain**: This helps to provide you with an overall healthy feeling by helping to calm your central nervous system, decongest the respiratory and live systems, cleanse toxins, helps with colds and coughs, and lower fevers. It provides the body with a calming effect. Research has found that this plant's leaves and flowers contain diuretic, antipyretic, and antispasmodic properties. Make sure that you only take a small dose of blue vervain because of its potency. If you take too much, it can induce vomiting and diarrhea.

- **Cancasa**: This is also called red willow bark, and helps to boost your libido.

- **Cascara Sagrada**: This amazing herb comes from the bark on the Rhamnus tree. The experts at the University of Michigan Health System think that the Native Americans began to use this herb in the 15th century, especially during the time when they showed the Spanish explorers its wonderful properties. They would use the plant as a laxative to help treat constipation. It can help soothe the large intestine's cells. Still today, over 20 percent of the national laxative market in the US depends on its properties.

- **Chaparral**: This herb is famous for curing the incurable. While you can get this herb in many different forms, the most commonly used form is dried. Herbalists will often use the dried herb in teas. It inhibits cancer cells from growing, nordihydroguaiaretic, and anti-tumor agents. It can also slow down cell proliferation and it prevents diseases from harming the DNA.

- **Cleavers**: This will purify the lymphatic system through its diuretic and tonic properties. It can also help to purify your body by healing conditions like psoriasis and arthritis. It can also help to clear out the urinary tract.

- **Contribo**: This herb has been noted for its use in Western Herbal Medicine. However, it can also be found in Ayurvedic medicine, as well as traditional Chinese medicine. Several different cultures throughout the world have used Contribo to treat various diseases. The ancient Byzantines, Romans, and Greeks would use it as part of their medicinal recipes to help treat lots of health problems. These experts would use the herb to help treat diseases like insomnia, uterine problems, snakebites, gout, bladder stones, and kidney ailments.

- **Dandelion**: Dandelion can help with eczema, gallstones, aching muscles, intestinal gas, loss of appetite, bruises, joint pain, and upset stomach. It is also good as a skin toner, and a digestive or blood tonic.

- **Damiana**: The damiana plant is a wild shrub. This has been a popular herbalist herb since the ancient Aztecs. This herb can be found in abundance in the West Indies, Central America, and Mexico, and is used to help various ailments. The natives in Mexico often use Damiana to boost their energy and improve their sexual potency. If you suffer from sexual problems, tension, nervousness, depression, or anxiety, this herb is the perfect herb for you.

- **Elderberry**: Elderberry can help with sciatica, sinus pain, neuralgia, and chronic fatigue syndrome. It can also be used to heal constipation, hay fever, and increase your flow of urine.

- **Eyebright**: Eyebright is also sometimes called Euphrasia and Meadow Eyebright. Researchers are working to prove its strength when it comes to helping treat visual disturbance, eye swelling, and eye redness. Eyebright can also relieve any eye issue that is caused by conjunctivitis and blepharitis. There are many different forms of eyebright. It can be found in powders, tablets, capsules, dried leaves, and in teabags.

- **Hydrangea**: Hydrangeas are not just an ornamental plant, but they are also a medicinal plant that is prevalent throughout North and South America, and Asia. The roots of the plant contain lots of nutrients and phytochemicals, such as selenium, zinc, and calcium. This makes them very important to herbalists because they can be used to treat lots of health problems. Some of the most common uses of hydrangeas are treating bladder and kidney diseases. Since the chemicals within the herb are able to increase urine output, it can help to treat urinary tract problems.

- **Irish Moss**: It is believed that Irish moss can provide nutrition on a cellular level. Some people also refer to Irish moss as sea moss, so these terms can be used interchangeably. Irish moss is very valuable for our health because it contains 92 out of 100 minerals that we have in our bodies. For this reason, Irish people have been known to rely on their health benefits in order to avoid starvation and to support their overall health. It has an exceptional nutritional profile. It contains 157 mg of phosphorus, 0.1 mg of copper, 0.5 mg of riboflavin, 144 mg of magnesium, and 8.9 mg of iron. It is also packed full of calcium, manganese, and zinc.

- **Lavender**: Lavender contains a lot of helpful properties, and this is what makes it a very important herb in the medical world. It contains linabol, flavonoids, triterpenoids, rosmarinic acid, camphor, borneol, cineole, and terpineol. When it is made into a balm, it is great for treating migraines and headaches.

- **Lily of the Valley**: This flowering plant flowers during late spring. It is most commonly found in the Northern Hemisphere in Europe and Asia. The leaves of the plant stand upright and are a glossy green color. They are able to reach a length of nine-inches and will reach a width of four inches. This flower contains a lot of properties. It works as a sedative, emetic, laxative, diuretic, and antispasmodic. Its effects are gradual, so it doesn't pose a threat to your kidneys.

- **Milk Thistle**: This can be helpful with liver conditions like jaundice, gallbladder disorders, cirrhosis, and hepatitis. Some even think it can help to lower cholesterol levels.

- **Nettles**: For centuries, nettles were used to help treat allergies. Dr. Andrew Wiel, who is the renowned author of *Natural Medicine,* states that when relieving allergy symptoms, he doesn't know anything that is as effective than nettle. Nettle has also shown promising signs in treating several other diseases, like prostate enlargement, bladder infections, asthma, arthritis, and Alzheimer's disease. Herbalists believe that the complete plant is very beneficial to the health of humans. This is why they use the leaves and stems when it comes to making medicines.

- **Prodigiosa**: This flowering plant is part of the daisy family. In some places throughout the world, it is referred to as the Mystical Caribbean, Love Leaf, and Arma poi. There are some who believe if you want to bring love into your life, all you have to do is write the name of the person you love on a piece of paper and lay a prodigiosa leaf over it. Besides that, if you have a lot of stress or suffer from headaches, you can place a couple of leaves over your head for a couple and minutes and it will ease your symptoms.

- **Red Clover**: This is used to help with various skin problems like eczema, psoriasis, sores, cancer, and burns. Red clover is a sedative, expectorant, antispasmodic, and deobstruent. Due to its properties, it has become one of Chile's economic staple. Many people will grow if for fodder, and it helps to replenish the fertility of the soil. Scientists have proven that clover also has a chemical called isoflavones that are similar to hormones. These important chemicals are nearly impossible to find in other herbs. They also have anti-inflammatory, antimicrobial, anticancer, and antioxidant properties.

- **Red Raspberry**: This has long been used to help pregnant women because it can help improve sleep, leg cramps, and counter nausea. It is high in iron, magnesium, B vitamins, and potassium.

- **Rhubarb Root**: This is a popular plant throughout the world. It has been used extensively in traditional Chinese medicines, by botanists, and Chinese herbalists. It is cultivated in large scales in China so that they can use it to treat serious health problems, such as digestive complaints and cancer. The roots also contain anthraquinones. This is a naturally occurring compound that has antioxidant, antiviral, antifungal, and antibacterial properties. All of these compounds are able to help protect you from malaria, kidney disease, liver disease, diabetes, and cancer.

- **Sage**: Ancient Greeks and Egyptians used sage to help treat bleeding, ulcers, swelling, and sprains. Many different lab tests that have been done have all confirmed all of its amazing nutritional value. A single tablespoon of sage contains 43 percent vitamin K. This is the amount that your body needs in order to work correctly. It is also a great source for magnesium, iron, calcium, vitamin E, vitamin A, vitamin C, and fiber. Researchers have also discovered that it also has B vitamins like riboflavin.

- **Santa Maria**: This plant is native to South and Central America, as well as Mexico. Studies have found that it holds quite a few health benefits. It is full of minerals and vitamins and holds several other key components such as camphor, sesquiterpene lactones, and volatile oil. All of these help the plant to treat problems like blood pressure, blood clots, migraines, inflammation, stress, anxiety, and arthritis.

- **Sarsaparilla Root**: This can help with the absorption of minerals because it is rich in iron. This plant can easily be found in warm, tropical areas all over the world. Sarsaparilla was used as herbal remedies for many thousands of years. This was a popular herb in Central and South America, and they used it to relieve quite a few problems. Herbalists have long used the powder of the roots in medicines that help treat the symptoms of joint pain, colds, headaches, and sexual impotence.

- **Valerian Root**: This is great for mild tremors, epilepsy, headaches, ADHS, depression, chronic fatigue syndrome, migraines, and upset stomach. It can also be helpful in fighting off insomnia.

- **Yellow Duck Root**: This can help with purifying the blood and detoxifying the liver. It can also trigger the bowel to help remove the waste that is in the intestinal tract and up your urine flow.

You can buy your own herbs and combine some of them to make your own infusions. An infusion is simply a tea. All you need is a reusable tea bag or ball. Steep your herb combination in some water that has boiled for at least five minutes and enjoy.

Stomach Soother

What you'll need:

- Agave syrup, 1 tbsp

- Ginger tea, .5 c

- Dr. Sebi's Stomach Relief Herbal Tea

- Burro banana, 1

What you'll do:

Fix the herbal tea according to the directions on the package. Set it aside to cool.

Once the tea is cool, place it along with all the other ingredients into a blender. Turn the blender on and let it run until it is creamy.

Sarsaparilla Syrup

What you'll need:

- Date sugar, 1 c
- Sassafras root, 1 tbsp
- Sarsaparilla root, 1 c
- Water, 2 c

What you'll do:

Start by adding all of the ingredients to a mason jar. Screw on the lid, tightly, and shake everything together. Heat a water bath up to 160. Sit the mason jar into the water bath and allow it to infuse for about two to four hours.

When the infusion time is almost up, set up an ice bath. Add half and half water and ice to a bowl. Carefully take the mason jar out of the water bath and place it into the ice bath. Allow it to sit in the ice bath for 15 to 20 minutes.

Strain the infusion out and into another clean jar. This will last for at least a week when kept in the refrigerator.

Dandelion "Coffee"

What you'll need:

- Nettle leaf, a pinch

- Roasted dandelion root, 1 tbsp

- Water, 24 oz

What you'll do:

To start, we will roast the dandelion root to help bring out its flavors. Feel free to use raw dandelion root if you want to, but roasted root brings out an earthy and complex flavor, which is perfect for cool mornings.

Simply add the dandelion root to a pre-warmed cast iron skillet. Allow the pieces to roast on medium heat until they start to darken in color, and you start to smell their rich aroma. Make sure that you don't let them burn because this will ruin your teas taste.

As the root is roasting, have the water in a pot and allow it to come up to a full, rapid boil. Once your dandelion is roasted, add it to the boiling water with the nettle leaf. Steep this for ten minutes.

Strain. You can flavor your tea with some agave if you want to. Enjoy.

Chamomile Delight

What you'll need:

- Date sugar, 1 tbsp

- Walnut milk, .5 c

- Dr. Sebi's Nerve/Stress Relief Herbal Tea, .25 c

- Burro banana, 1

What you'll do:

Prepare the tea according to the package directions. Set to the side and allow to cool.

Once the tea is cooled, add it along with the above ingredients to a blender and process until creamy and smooth.

Mucus Cleanse Tea

What you'll need:

- Blue Vervain

- Bladderwrack

- Irish Sea Moss

What you'll do:

Add the sea moss to your blender. This would be best as a gel. Just make sure that it is totally dry.

Place equal parts of the bladderwrack to the blender. Again this would be best as a gel. Just make sure that it is totally dry. To get the best results you need to chop these by hand.

Add equal parts of the blue vervain to the blender. You can use the roots to increase your iron intake and nutritional healing values.

Process the herbs until they form a powder. This can take up to three minutes.

Place the powder into a non-metal pot and put it on the stove. Fill the pot half full of water. Make sure the herbs are totally immersed in water. Turn on the heat and let the liquid boil. Don't let it boil more than five minutes.

Carefully strain out the herbs. You can save these for later use in other recipes.

Let the liquid cool to your liking and enjoy.

You can add in some agave nectar, date sugar, or key lime juice for added flavor.

ImmuniTea

What you'll need:

- Echinacea, 1 part
- Astragalus, 1 part
- Rosehip, 1 part
- Chamomile, 1 part
- Elderflowers, 1 part
- Elderberries, 1 part

What you'll do:

Mix the herbs together and place them inside an airtight container.

When you are ready to make a cup of tea, place one teaspoon into a tea ball or bag, and put it in eight ounces of boiling water. Let this sit for 20 minutes.

Ginger Turmeric Tea

What you'll need:

- Juice of one key lime
- Turmeric finger, couple of slices
- Ginger root, couple of slices
- Water, 3 c

What you'll do:

Pour the water into a pot and let it boil. Remove from heat and put the turmeric and ginger in. Stir well. Place lid on pot and let it sit 15 minutes.

While you are waiting on your tea to finish steeping, juice one key lime, and divide between two mugs.

Once the tea is ready, remove the turmeric and ginger and pour the tea into mugs and enjoy. If you want your tea a bit sweet, add some agave syrup or date sugar.

Tranquil Tea

What you'll need:

- Rose petals, 2 parts
- Lemongrass, 2 parts
- Chamomile, 4 parts

What you'll do:

Put all the herbs into a glass jar and shake well to mix.

When you are ready to make a cup of tea, add one teaspoon of the mixture for every serving to a tea strainer, ball, or bag. Cover with water that has boiled and let it sit for ten minutes.

If you like a little sweetness in your tea, you can add some agave syrup or date sugar.

Energizing Lemon Tea

What you'll need:

- Lemongrass, .5 tsp. dried herb

- Lemon thyme, .5 tsp. dried herb

- Lemon verbena, 1 tsp. dried herb

What you'll do:

Place the dried herbs into a tea strainer, bag, or ball and place it in one cup of water that has boiled. Let this sit 15 minutes. Carefully strain out the tea. You can add agave syrup or date sugar if needed.

Quick note: If your herbs are fresh, you just need to triple the amounts above.

Pregnan-Tea

What you'll need:

- Nettle leaf, 1 c
- Stevia leaf, .25 c
- Ginger root, two inches
- Raspberry leaf, 4 cups

What you'll do:

Mix all of the above together and store in a glass jar.

When you are ready for a cup of tea, place one tablespoon into a cup of water that has boiled. Let this sit for ten minutes. If you need it a bit sweeter, add more stevia leaves or agave syrup.

If you would like to make this by the gallon to have on hand, place one cup of the ingredients into one gallon of water that has boiled let it sit for 20 minutes. Keep on hand in the refrigerator.

This tea is great to drink during pregnancy as it helps with digestive and nausea problems. It also strengthens the uterus. Nettle gives the body vitamin K which is essential for birth and pregnancy to help with clotting.

Most women have reported that they actually have faster and easier labors after using this tea. This is a delicious tea to drink at any time but it is very helpful during pregnancy.

Respiratory Support Tea

What you'll need:

- Rosehip, 2 parts
- Lemon balm, 1 part
- Coltsfoot leaves, 1 part
- Mullein, 1 part
- Osha root, 1 part
- Marshmallow root, 1 part

What you'll do:

Place three cups of water into a pot. Place the Osha root and marshmallow root into the pot. Allow to boil. Let this simmer for ten minutes

Now put the remaining ingredients into the pot and let this steep another eight minutes. Strain.

Drink three to four cups of this tea each day.

It's almost that time of year again when everyone is suffering from the dreaded cold. Then that cold turns into a nasty lingering cough. Having these ingredients on hand will help you be able to get ahead of this year's cold season. When you buy your ingredient, they need to be stored in glass jars. The roots and leaves need to be put into separate jars. You can drink this tea at any time, but it is great for when you need some extra respiratory support.

Thyme and Lemon Tea

What you'll need:

- Key lime juice, 2 tsp.

- Fresh thyme sprigs, 2

What you'll do:

Place the thyme into a canning jar. Boil enough water to cover the thyme sprigs. Cover the jar with a lid and leave it alone for ten minutes. Add the key lime juice. Carefully strain into a mug and add some agave nectar if desired.

This tea is great for easing cold and cough symptoms and calming a sore throat.

Sore Throat Tea

What you'll need:

- Sage leaves, 8 to 10 leaves

What you'll do:

Place the sage leaves into a quart canning jar and add water that has boiled until it covers the leaves. Put the lid on the jar and let sit for 15 minutes.

You can use this tea as a gargle to help ease a sore or scratchy throat. Usually, the pain will ease up before you even finish your first cup. This can also be used for inflammations of the throat, tonsils, and mouth since the mucous membranes get soothed by the sage oil. A normal dose would be between three to four cups each day. Every time you take a sip, roll it around in your mouth before swallowing it.

If you like to garden, you might have some sage on hand. Just cut some leaves during the summer and fall to make sure you have a decent supply of dried leaves at all times. If you must, you can get some at your grocery store or local market.

Autumn Tonic Tea

What you'll need:

- Dried ginger root, 1 part

- Rosehip, 1 part

- Red clover, 2 parts

- Dandelion root and leaf, 2 parts

- Mullein leaf, 2 parts

- Lemon balm, 3 parts

- Nettle leaf, 4 parts

What you'll do:

Place all of these ingredients above into a bowl. Stir everything together to mix well. Put into a glass jar with a lid and keep it in a dry place that stays cool.

When you want a cup of tea, place four cups of water into a pot. Let this come to a full rolling boil. Place the desired amount of tea blend into a tea strainer, ball, or bag and cover with boiling water. Let sit for 15 minutes. Strain out the herbs and drink it either cold or hot. If you like your tea sweet, add some agave syrup or date sugar.

Adrenal and Stress Health

What you'll need:

- Bladderwrack, .5 c
- Tulsi holy basil, 1 c
- Shatavari root, 1 c
- Ashwagandha root, 1 c

What you'll do:

Place these ingredients into a bowl. Stir well to combine.

Place mixture in a glass jar with a lid and store in a dry place that stays cool.

When you want a cup of tea, place two tablespoons of the tea mixture into a medium pot. Pour in two cups of water. Let this come to a full rolling boil. Turn down heat. Let this simmer 20 minutes. Strain well. If you like your tea sweet, you can add some agave syrup or date sugar.

Lavender Tea

What you'll need:

- Agave syrup, to taste
- Dried lavender flowers, 2 tbsp
- Fresh lemon balm, handful
- Water, 3 c

What you'll do:

Pour the water in a pot and allow to boil.

Pour over the lavender and lemon balm. Cover and let sit for five minutes.

Strain well. If you like your tea sweet, add some agave syrup.

This tea is great for any time of the day, but it's great at night since it does help you relax.

Rosy Black Tea

What you'll need:

- Black tea, 1 part

- Rose petals, 2 parts

What you'll do:

Put the black tea and rose petals into a glass jar. Shake vigorously until well mixed.

When you are ready to make tea, put one teaspoon into a tea strainer, bag, or ball. Place into your most favorite mug and pour water that has boiled over it. Let this sit for five minutes. Take the tea strainer out and add some agave syrup if you want something a bit sweeter.

Tranquil Tea

What you'll need:

- Rose petals, 2 parts

- Lemongrass, 2 parts

- Chamomile, 4 parts

What you'll do:

Place the herbs into a glass jar and shake vigorously until well combined.

When you are ready for a cup of tea, place one teaspoon of the tea blend into a mug and add eight ounces of boiling water. Let sit between five and ten minutes.

If you like your tea sweet, add some agave syrup or date sugar.

Soothing Lemon Tea

What you'll need:

- Stevia leaf, pinch
- Chamomile, .25 c
- Lemon peel, .25 c
- Lemon balm, .25 c
- Lemongrass, .75 c

What you'll do:

Place all the above ingredients into a glass jar and shake vigorously to combine well.

When you are ready to have a cup of tea, take one teaspoon of the tea and put it into a tea ball, bag, or strainer. Put this into your favorite mug and cover with a cup of water that has boiled.

Let this sit for five minutes. If you want your tea sweeter, you can add more stevia leaf or agave syrup.

Morning Refresher

What you'll need:

- Boiling water, 2 c

- Dried lavender, .5 tsp.

- Fennel seeds, 1 tsp.

- Dried rosebuds, 3 to 5

- Fresh fennel, 5 sprigs

What you'll do:

Place the herbs in your teapot or in a cup. Pour in the boiling water. Allow everything to sit and steep for three to five minutes. Strain the tea mixture out of the tea and enjoy.

Berry Lime Tea

What you'll need:

- Boiling water, 2 c

- Dried lime peel, 2 tsp.

- Juniper berries, 2 tsp.

What you'll do:

Add the lime peel and berries to a teapot or glass. Cover them with water that has boiled and let them sit five minutes. If you want a stronger flavor, you can allow them to steep longer. Strain the tea mixture out and enjoy.

Zestea

What you'll need:

- Boiling water, 2 c

- Dried lime peel, 2 tsp.

- Fennel seeds, 2 tsp.

What you'll do:

Add the fennel seeds and lime peel to a teapot or a cup. Cover them with the boiling water. Allow the tea to steep for at least five minutes. The longer you let it steep, the stronger the tea will be. Strain the tea mixture out and enjoy.

Feminine Balance Tea

What you'll need:

- All of the ingredients below are dried
- Vitex, 1 c
- Hibiscus flowers, 1 c
- Orange peel, 1 c
- Lemon balm, 1 c
- Rose petals, 1 c
- Fennel seeds, 1 c
- Oatstraw, 1 c
- Yarrow, 1 c
- Nettle, 1 c
- Raspberry leaf, 1 c
- Red clover leaf, 1 c
- Red clover blossoms, 1 c
- Alfalfa, 1 c

What you'll do:

Place all of the ingredients listed above into a bowl and stir well to combine. Store in a glass jar in a cool, dark place.

When you are ready for a cup of tea, use one teaspoon of the herbs for every cup of water. Pour water that has boiled over the tea and steep for 20 minutes. If you want a more potent infusion, you can let it sit for up to eight hours.

You can sweeten the tea by adding some agave nectar or date sugar.

You can drink a quart of this each day, either room temperature or warm.

In order to get the most benefits from this tea, you need to drink one quart of this each day. It will give you a boost of energy and can help with nourishment, balancing anxiety, and mood, along with other benefits.

DO NOT take it during pregnancy.

Pregnancy-Safe Headache Tea

What you'll need:

- Lemon peel, 1 c
- Lavender, 1 c
- Lemon balm, 1 c
- Skullcap, 1 c
- Chamomile, 1 c

What you'll do:

Place all the above ingredients into a large bowl and combine well. Place into a glass jar and keep in a dark place that stays cool.

When you are ready for a cup of tea, put one to two teaspoons of the tea mix into one cup of boiling water. Make sure to put the tea into a tea strainer, bag, or ball.

Allow the tea to steep for at least 15 minutes. If you like your tea sweet, you can add some agave syrup or date sugar.

Drink either cold or hot when you feel a headache beginning.

Getting a headache when you are breastfeeding or pregnant can be tough because normal OTC medicines won't work. Eating something might help. Think about what you have eaten during the day because a headache could mean that you are deficient in something like magnesium.

Headaches could be brought on by fatigue, stress, or weather. A cup of tea could help nourish your body while getting rid of some stress and letting you get some much-needed rest. You need to use caution when breastfeeding or pregnant, as some herbs can be harmful to newborn fetuses. If you have a history of miscarriages, you will need to do some research especially during the first trimester.

The herbs above are all fine to be used during breastfeeding and pregnancy. If you are unsure, do some research. Always use your best judgment.

Teething Tea

What you'll need:

- Cloves, .5 c
- Red clover, 5 c
- Rosehip, 5 c
- Oatstraw, .5 c
- Skullcap, .5 c
- Catnip, 5 c
- Lavender, .5 c
- Chamomile, .5 c

What you'll do:

Place all the above herbs into a glass jar and shake well to combine. Keep the jar in a dark place that stays cool.

When you want a cup of tea, place two teaspoons of the dried herbs into one cup of water. Allow to sit for 20 minutes. If you want a more potent infusion, you can let it sit for four hours or overnight. You can let your child drink it either a bit warm or chilled.

You could even place a washcloth into the tea and wring it out. Place the cloth in the freezer and your child can chew on the cloth when needed.

Ginger Shot

What you'll need:

- Small apple

- Fresh ginger root, 2 oz

What you'll do:

Get rid of the skin on the ginger. Using a spoon is an easier option. Once peeled, chop it, and add it to your juicer.

Slice up your apples and add them in with the ginger. Juice them together, and enjoy.

You could just use a blender if you don't have access to a juicer. When using a blender, you will add the ginger and apple along with one to two cups of spring water. Blend everything together, and then strain it through some cheesecloth. Enjoy.

Rose Tea Jam

What you'll need:

- Sea moss gel, 4 tbsp
- Date sugar, 4 c
- Zest of a lime
- Juice of a lime
- Peach
- Apple
- Mango
- Currants, .5 c
- Pear
- Chopped rose hips, .25 c
- Rose petals, 1 c
- Hibiscus flowers, 6 whole flowers
- Water, 8 c

What you'll do:

Start by washing, coring, and cutting the fruit into quarter-inch pieces. Using kitchen scissors, carefully cut the hibiscus flowers.

Add the water, hibiscus, and rosehips to a pot and allow everything to come up to a boil. At the same time, in another pot, add the remaining water and the sugar and let them come to a boil.

Let both pots of water to boil for three minutes and make sure you stir then often. Set them off of the heat and add the rose petals into the hibiscus tea you created. Add in the fresh chopped fruit to the pot of sugar water. Stir in vigorously for about a minute.

Let both of the pots cool for around five minutes. You can let them sit a bit longer if you want the flavor to be stronger. At this point, you can filter the flowers out of the tea if you want.

In a glass bowl that can hold upwards of ten cups, pour in both pots of water. Mix in the lime extra and lime juice, stirring until completely mixed together. Stir in the sea moss gel.

Make sure you have glass jars that have been sterilized in the boiling water.

Scoop the jam mixture into the jars, leaving about a quarter of an inch space at the top. Clean the rims and screw on the lids. At this point, you can simple freeze or refrigerate, or you can complete the canning process.

To can them completely, place them in a pot of boil water so that they are completely covered. Let them boil for ten minutes. Let them rest for another ten minutes before you try to take the jars out of the water. Remove the jars with jar tongs and let them sit to the side until they cool off completely. While they are still hot, if anything cold hits them, they can explode. Make sure you label your jars. This jam will probably not be as thick as the jams you are used to.

Ginger Tea

What you'll need:

- Raw agave
- Pinch of cayenne
- Lime juice, 2 tbsp
- Fresh dill weed, 1 to 2 sprigs
- Ginger root, 1 thumb
- Springwater, 4 c

What you'll do:

Allow some water to come to a full rolling boil.

Peel your ginger and then chop. Put it in your boiling water with the dill. Let this boil for about five minutes.

Strain your tea into a glass jar.

Mix in the lime juice.

Stir in the agave and cayenne to taste.

This can be enjoyed cold or hot.

Sea Moss/Irish Moss Gel

What you'll need:

- Spring water, 1.5 to 2 c

- Sea moss, 1 c

What you'll do:

Work through your sea moss, rinsing and cleaning it, and inspecting for sand and any other debris, before continuing. Once you are done cleaning the sea moss, allow it to soak in water for four to 24 hours at room temp. Make sure that you change the water every four to six hours.

Once the sea moss is done soaking, it will be white-translucent in color. It is also going to be slippery and soft. It will have doubled in size. Drain all of the water off and rinse it clean.

Place the moss and the spring water to your blender and mix them together until they are smooth and creamy.

Pour into a glass, lidded jar, and keep it refrigerated. It will take about an hour before it thickens up. You can use this in any recipe that calls for sea moss or sea moss gel.

Stinging Nettle Tea

What you'll need:

- Fresh or dry nettle leaves, 3 tbsp

- Ginger, 2 slices

- Agave syrup

What you'll do:

Add the ginger and nettle to a French Press or into a quart jar. Cover the herbs with hot water and allow them to sit and steep for at least 20 minutes. You can let it steep overnight if you would like a strong infusion.

Once you are ready to enjoy, stir in agave syrup if you feel it needs to be sweetened, and enjoy.

Relaxing Rose Tea

What you'll need:

- Blue cornflowers, .75 c

- Rose petals, .75 c

- Lemon balm, .75 c

- Chamomile, 1 c

- Fennel, .25 c

- Tila, 2 c

What you'll do:

To start, we will mix the herbal blend together. Add all of the herbs and flowers to a large, lidded bowl and mix them together. As long as it is covered, it should last for a month.

To make hot tea, add a teaspoon of the tea mixture to a cup and add water that has boiled. Allow everything to sit for five to 15 minutes. Strain the tea out. You can sweeten it with agave if you want.

To make brewed iced tea, you will add two tablespoons of the tea mixture into a quart jar and cover the herbs with boiling water. Allow this to steep for 15 minutes. Strain. Pour into a larger jar, mix in some agave if you want and then mix in two cups of cold water. Enjoy.

Conclusion

Thank you for making it through to the end of *Dr. Sebi Recipe Book*, let's hope it was informative and able to provide you with all of the tools you need to achieve your goals whatever they may be.

The next step is to start trying out these recipes that are within this book. You can always transition into Dr. Sebi's diet if switching straight to it might be too much. That is perfectly okay. You do what feels best for your body. Dr. Sebi's diet is supposed to help you feel better. The best first step is to head to the grocery store and purchase the foods you need for Dr. Sebi's diet. There's a good chance you already have some of them. Above all, enjoy these recipes, and know that when you are eating them, you are feeding your body with the nutrients that it wants and needs.

Finally, if you found this book useful in any way, a review on Amazon is always appreciated!

Description

Have you learned about Dr. Sebi's diet and ready to get started? Can't figure out what to cook? Well, you don't have to look any further. Continue reading, and you'll learn why.

Dr. Sebi's alkaline diet can turn your unhealthy body into a health machine. Dr. Sebi learned that modern medicine wasn't curing diseases, but, instead, was creating more problems for people. He learned about herbalism from his grandmother and an herbalist in Mexico and realized that this was the key to a much better health. Through the herbalist in Mexico, he was able to heal all the health problems that he had been diagnosed with.

This is where Dr. Sebi's diet was born. He learned that if you made sure that the body stayed in an alkaline state, diseases couldn't thrive. Diseases need acid in order to live and grow. While his diet will require you to cut out a lot of foods, a lot of people have found success with his teachings. This book is here to provide you recipes to help you get started on Dr. Sebi's diet. All of the recipes follow his nutrition guide so that you know you are eating nothing but approved foods. The only thing you will need to do is decide on what supplements you need to take.

Within this book, you will find:

- Introduction to Dr. Sebi's diet

- How to use Dr. Sebi's diet of natural eating to become healthy

- The best alkaline meals that you can enjoy throughout the day

- Delicious smoothies that will nourish and heal your body

- Herb recipes that will leave you feeling good and healthy

- Over 100+ easy and tasty meals to prepare

- A wide variety of teas that will aid your daily health issues like

  - Respiratory Support Teas

  - Pregnancy Teas

  - Energizing Teas

  - Stomach soothing Teas

  - Teething Teas

  - Stress Teas

  - Pregnancy-Safe Headache Tea

  - AND MORE

- A delicious selection of smoothies, desserts, cereals, wraps & sandwiches, pasta & pizza, soups, and salads

... And so much more.

This book does not skimp on recipes either. Within these pages, you will find 100+ different recipes. You will find that the ingredients needed are all super easy to find. You don't need processed foods or a bunch of additives to make tasty meals. Foods in their natural state taste delicious on their own.

Diet doesn't have to be complicated. Dr. Sebi makes your diet simple, effective, and worthwhile. If you are serious about your health, then choosing this book will be one of the best decisions you will ever make. Chances are, you are already aware of Dr. Sebi, and you are looking for an easy way to get started. Even if you aren't sure who he is, this book will lead you in the right direction.

If you pass on this book, you will regret it. Make the right decision to change your life for the better. Get this book today and start trying out these delicious recipes. Scroll up and click "buy now" right now.

Extra content: Explore the collection of books about Dr. Sebi

I wrote this collection in order to reach as many people as possible the knowledge of Dr. Sebi. Do a lot of studies and extract all the information that can lead a person to experience a real change in their life, in a simple way. Here is a preview of what you will find in the rest of the books and you will be able to empirically experience the benefits of following his teachings in a complete way.

Dr. Sebi Treatment and Cures Book:

Dr. Sebi Cure for STDs, Herpes, HIV, Diabetes, Lupus, Hair Loss, Kidney, and Other Diseases

Table of Contents

Introduction

"A healthy body is worth more than any dollar amount. You don't want to be the wealthiest person on a hospital bed." – Dr. Sebi

Congratulations on taking the first steps to improve your health by choosing Dr. Sebi Treatment and Cures Book. In this book, you will learn all of the healing secrets of Dr. Sebi and how they can help you to improve your health.

Throughout this book, we will discuss the various treatment methods laid out by Dr. Sebi to help you recover from STDs, diabetes, hair loss, lupus, and kidney disease. But before we jump into that information, let's take a look at who Dr. Sebi is.

"Healing has to be consistent with life itself. If it isn't, then it is not healing. The components have to be from life." – Dr. Sebi

Dr. Sebi was born as Alfredo Darrington Bowman on November 26, 1933, in Illanga, Honduras. His grandmother taught him about herbal healing. He was self-educated. Dr. Sebi is considered a naturalist, biochemist, herbalist, and pathologist. Over his years, he studied herbs all over North, Central, and South America, Caribbean, and Africa. He developed and unique methodology and approach to healing humans with herbs that are rooted in more than 30 years of experience.

When he moved to the US, he wasn't happy with the modern medical practices that they used to treat things like impotency, diabetes, and asthma. He had been diagnosed with obesity, impotence, diabetes, and asthma, and had undergone many modern medical treatments that did not help him. That's what led him to an herbalist in Mexico, and shortly thereafter, he started his herbal healing practice in New York.

He eventually started a second practice, which he called the USHA Research Institute, in La Ceiba, Honduras. He worked with many well-known celebrities, including Michael Jackson, Eddie Murphy, John Travolta, Steven Seagal, and Lisa Lopes.

Dr. Sebi dedicated more than 30 years of his life to come up with a methodology that he was only able to come up with through years of empirical knowledge. Inspired by all of his own healing knowledge and experience he had learned, he started to share the compounds with other people. This is how he gave birth to Dr. Sebi's Cell Food.

Dr. Sebi passed away on August 9, 2016, from pneumonia.

"Growth is painful, change is painful, but nothing is as painful as staying the same." – Dr. Sebi

Dr. Sebi Food List Recipes:

The Real 7-Day-Detox Method Cleanse with Approved Foods Following a Step-by-Step Dr. Sebi Alkaline Diet

Table of Contents

Conclusion

Introduction

First off, I would like to congratulate you for choosing *Dr. Sebi Food List Recipes* and taking a huge leap towards optimal health. Dr. Sebi was an amazing herbalist and naturalist, and has shown many people the best way to reach amazing health.

While there may be many people out there who don't understand Dr. Sebi, there are just as many who know that his teachings are helpful. If this is the first time you have ever heard of Dr. Sebi, let me take a moment to introduce you to him.

Dr. Sebi was born in Honduras as Alfredo Bowman. He was a self-taught man, and studied herbs all over the Americas and Africa. While he was taught about herbs from his grandmother at a young age, it was when he moved to America that he really dove into his studies.

Once in America, he was diagnosed with several diseases, but none of the remedies helped. That is when he went to an herbalist in Mexico. He saw great success with the herbalist, and this inspired his Dr. Sebi's Cell Food. Through the years he has helped many people, along with some celebrities.

This book is here to present to you Dr. Sebi's 7-day detox. This will help to reset your body and prepare it for a healthy future. Throughout the book, you will learn about Dr. Sebi's food list, his 10 commandments, and how to prepare yourself for the detox.

The great thing is, you can take the food list and continue to follow Dr. Sebi's diet after you have finished the detox. You will also feel amazing and your body will be thanking your for making it healthier.

Disclaimer

Please note that we are not doctors and we do not claim to be. We simply follow the instructions of Dr. Sebi.

Chapter 1: Before You Begin

There are many different types of cleanses, from fasting to whole-foods, but they all aim to accomplish the same thing, and that is to get rid of inflammatory substances and toxicity. Then they provide your body with pure forms of nutrients. The goal of a cleanse is to heal and restore your body to its optimal health, and give its powerful detoxification systems to work without the blockages that are normally there.

The occasional detox is great for the body, but you should never just jump straight into a detox. Getting your body ready for the detox is just as important as the actual detox. If you already follow a very healthy and clean diet, then you won't have as much to do to get ready. But if you are like most people and follow a standard American diet, then you will have some work to do.

Cleanse and detox are words that tend to be used interchangeably, but they aren't quite the same thing. A cleanse is something that you do that will cause detoxification. Your body detoxes naturally as soon as your food has been digesting. This is where it will remove toxic and foreign materials. Unfortunately, the regular lifestyle and diets of most people causes them to accumulate more toxins than the body is able to purge. Because of this, we need to, on occasion, do a cleanse or fast where we consciously reduce the number of toxins that we are consuming so that the body is forced into a natural detoxifying state.

A cleanse could be a complete abstinence from food or toxic activities, and you only consume water. This type of fast might be helpful, but it's pretty hard to keep up. The Dr. Sebi detox won't require you to stop eating altogether, but if you want to try that type of cleanse, feel free to because it can do amazing things to your body.

Starting just a few days before you plan on beginning your detox, you will want to start changing how you eat. You will need to eat simple, light foods like salads, soups, or veggies. You will want to focus on raw veggies and leafy greens. This is especially true if you haven't been much of a clean eater. You need to give you body a chance to get ready for the cleanse. Take little steps by slowly cutting out processed and sugar foods, and star to increase you intake of fresh foods and grains.

Taking these small steps will increase your body's alkalinity to help it get ready for the deeper cleanse of your detox. During the detox, your body is going to end up releasing toxins that are stored in your tissues. These toxins may enter your bloodstream and can end up causing trouble sleeping, mood swings, body odor, bad breath, aches and pains, or rashes. By preparing for your detox, you can minimize your chances of developing these side effects.

To help you out, we will go over some tips on getting your body ready for your detox.

Dietary Changes

- Begin Your Day Right

You should start adding in a glass of warm lime water to your daily routine. This helps to jump-start your digestion and boost your metabolism. Lime juice is very alkalizing to your body, rich in vitamin C, and helps to cleanse your liver, which are all very important parts of detoxification.

- Switch Up Your Drinks

You will want to start drinking more spring water during the day, and start adding in some cleansing herbal teas, such as burdock, dandelion root, or nettle tea. This is also the best time to switch from regular tap water to spring water. You have to drink spring water while on Dr. Sebi's detox.

If you drink alcohol or coffee, you need to start cutting back on your consumption of them. You won't be able to have them on the detox. To let go of coffee, a good alternative is herbal or green tea. While green tea does contain caffeine, it is full of antioxidants, which will help your detoxification. Sodas and energy drinks should also be eliminated.

Water will play a very big part in your life, so beginning your day with two glasses of water is helpful in getting ready for your detox. If you choose to do the hot lime water, that counts towards a glass.

- Keep Things Simple

Start to change you meals to something that is very simple and easy to make. You should opt for dishes that are heavy in natural fruits and vegetables and start weaning yourself off of meats, if you are a meat eater. Include a lot of foods that are rich in chlorophyll because these aid in detoxification.

This can also include drinking veggie soups and broths. If you find it hard to eat enough vegetables, you can get your veggie intake through smoothies or juice. An easy way to add more fruits and veggies into your current diet is by adding a piece of organic fresh fruit to your breakfast each morning. You can also turn to fresh fruits as your mid-afternoon snack instead of heading to the vending machine. When picking out your fruits and veggies, go with organic, seasonal, and local produce when you can so that you avoid pesticides.

- Reduce Your Animal Product Intake

You are going to have to cut out animal products completely on Dr. Sebi's fast, so leading up to it, you should start weaning yourself off of them. The first place to start is to stop eating processed and red meats. This includes things like cured meats and sausages. Choosing leaner meats and fish is a better choice during this time. When picking fish, stay away from fish that are high in mercury, like mackerel and tuna. Fish like salmon, scallops, anchovies, and shrimp are better options.

- Check Your Oils

A lot of people will cook with vegetable or canola oil because the health industry tells you they are better because they are lower in fat, but they aren't. You need to start using olive oil, avocado oil, coconut oil, and grapeseed oil. Coconut and olive oils should not be cooked and should only be used raw. You can also use these oils along with some lime juice and herbs to create your own salad dressings.

- Up Your Grain Intake

Right now, you don't have to worry about eating Dr. Sebi approved grains. All you need to worry about is increasing how much whole grains you eat. Start eating more brown rice or spelt, and also start eating more pseudo-grains like quinoa. You need to start reducing how much refined foods like pasta and bread you consume, and that includes whole-grain bread or pasta. Do your best to avoid wheat wherever you are able to.

- Get Rid of Refined Sugar

You have to start reading nutrition levels to make sure that foods aren't hiding sugars. Before the detox, you can pick healthier sugar alternatives in moderation. Maple syrup, raw honey, rapadura sugar, coconut blossom syrup, coconut sugar, or agave nectar are great alternatives. Once the detox starts, you will only be able to have agave nectar.

- Get Rid of Table Salt

Table salt does not provide you with any nutrients. Your body also has a very hard time metabolizing table salt. While you are checking nutrition labels for sugars, check and make sure they aren't hiding any table salts. The majority of processed foods will have large amounts of chemically processed salts. You should use sea salt as your salt source. It is full of minerals and they are able to help get rid of heavy metals within your body.

- Cut Out Unhealthy Foods

Leading up to the detox, you should slowly start cutting out unhealthy foods that you like to eat. This includes things like store-bought cookies or muffins, chips, and fried foods. Choose, instead, to snack on homemade dried fruit, seeds, and unsalted nuts. Before the detox, feel free to try some raw chocolate to help you with your chocolate fix.

Get Your Mind Ready

But what should we do about the mind? There is a lot of evidence that has found that our mental state, from stressed to relaxed and all that is in between, has a large impact on our wellbeing and health. While you can do a cleanse for a week without changing anything else about your day, and you may feel pretty good after, but, when you add mindfulness into your cleanse, you will uncovering some amazing opportunities to move your focus inwards to create as much space in your emotional body and mind as you can in the physical body.

You could possibly be at a time of transition and you're looking for a fresh start to push yourself into the next phase. You could be holding onto something, such as a loss, fear, resentment, or unhealthy relationship, that you want to get rid of. Maybe most of your day is spent focusing on and caring for other people and feel like you need to do something for yourself. A lot of use resist turning in, and may even fear it. You could have an inner voice asking you to stop distracting yourself in order to listen to your intuition.

In order to get the most from your cleanse, it is a good idea to like what you want to get rid of other than the junk in your diet, and why you are drawn to this cleanse.

- Relax And Meditate

Getting ready for the cleanse doesn't just mean getting your belly ready for the change in foods, but it also means making sure your mind is ready for the change. Relaxation and mediation are a big part of detoxing because they can help you to reduce or eliminate your stress. Stress is the number one cause of so many unhealthy habits, such snacking on junk food or overeating. If you simply set aside some time each day to simple sit and be still, it will help to quiet your mind. This will help you to remain focused on what your goals are.

- Start Journalling

It's also a good idea to start keeping a detox journal. While you are getting ready for your detox, you can take the time to write out the guidelines for it, or simply write out what you hope it will do for you. In it, you should also make sure you schedule rest time. Your body will be doing a lot of work, and it's common to start feeling tired. Making sure you have rest time set aside will help to combat any fatigue you may experience. While detoxing, you can expel mental toxins by writing in the journal. You can write anything you want so that you mentally cleanse yourself. Let the words flow and don't worry if it makes sense, is grammatically correct, or what have you. Simply writing things out on paper is very therapeutic.

- Clear Your Space

While this might not seem important, but before you start cleaning your insides, you should also clean your outside. It has been proven that the health of mind is greatly impacted by your surroundings and all of the environmental toxins lurking in your space. Take the time to vacuum the floor, give your sheets a change, and use an air filter. You should also create your own sanctuary that you can use during your cleanse. This could be an entire room in your house, if you have a spare one, or it could simply be a comfy chair placed next to a window. Wherever you place your sanctuary, remove all of the clutter and place a vase of some of your favorite flowers or simply a photo that makes you happy. You can also choose something that calms or inspires you.

- Let Your Family and Friends Know

You are getting ready to embark on something that is likely going to be very different from your everyday life. That means, anybody you socialize with on a regular basis is probably going to notice something. Those that you live with will definitely notice something. To make sure that you are successful at your cleanse you will want to let your inner circle know what you are doing. Make sure that you get everybody on the same page so that they will know why you can't do certain things or go out to certain places during your weeklong cleanse. Your closest friends and family tend to be your biggest cheerleaders, so they may just be the person you turn to when you feel like giving up.

That being said, don't be surprised if you one of them question you about your choice of cleanse. If this happens, simply explain to them why you want to do this. If that's not good enough for them, don't try to change their mind. You don't have to have their approval to do this. You are doing this only for you, and not for them. If you have to keep your distance from them during the cleanse, then do so. Do what is best for you.

- Change Up Your Inner Dialogue

You know all of the negativity that tends to be swarming around in your head? You know that defeatist inner monologue that everybody tends to slip into from time to time? Now, is all of that serving you at all? When you start telling yourself that you aren't good enough, smart enough, skinny enough, and so, does it help you reach your goals? It is now time for you to change that inner dialogue. What though patterns will you be able to let go of as you are cleansing? To help you out, try writing down the negative things that you have told yourself. Underneath that negative thought, in bigger letters, change that negative sentence into a positive one. Things like "I can do anything I set my mind to," "I am worthy," or "I am beautiful the way I am" are all great choices. You should also think about making this your mantra for your cleanse. You should say this out loud each and every day. At first, you might not believe the words coming out of your mouth, but after awhile, you will start to believe it.

- Pick a Good Time

While there likely is no perfect time to do a detox, it's a good idea to look at your calendar to see when you have the most free time. If you do, by chance, of a week of vacation built up at work and haven't made any other plans that might be a good option that way you don't have to worry about work. It's also a good idea to make sure that you detox won't occur during any major life events, holidays, important projects at work, or vacations. You definitely don't want to have a marathon run scheduled during the time you plan on doing your detox. It is just for a week, so it shouldn't be too hard to find at least one week where you don't have a lot going on.

- Think About a Digital Detox

This isn't something that you have to do, but it might be a good option if you are able to. Try to go digital-free for at least one whole day during your cleanse. The majority of people carry incredible power around with us in the form of tiny computers in your pocket. Remember, this cleanse that you have planned is time that you have set aside for yourself in order to remove junk from your life and replenish you system with healthy things.

This is true for your mind just as much as it is for your entire body. When you are going to the gym or heading out somewhere, leave your phone at home. Switch off your social media notifications. Choose one or two hours during the day to go through your emails or create an away message to let people know that you will get back to them tomorrow. Now that you have carved out some undistracted time, do something fun or healthy, like reading a book, write a letter, take a walk, or work on that project you have been meaning to for months. Whatever you want to do, that doesn't have to do with the digital world, do it.

- Lean Into Your Breath

When you start to experience the emotional or physical side effects of the cleanse, take a few minutes to simply breath so that you can connect with your body. This will help to slow your heart rate, help you to deal with imagined or real hunger, push through your erratic energy or mood swing, and then move the focus on your mind back into focus.

To do this, all you need to do is either stand or sit still and let your eyes close gently, or leave them open if you need to. Then take ten deep breaths in through your nose and release them out your mouth. As you inhale, picture it as a cleansing energy and view your exhale as a release of negativity. This can easily be done anywhere, like sitting in traffic or at the grocery store. Simply moving your attention to the movement of your breath will help to bring you into the present moment.

- Find a Cleanse Buddy

This might not be possible, but see if you can create some support for yourself and find somebody to do the cleanse with you. While a week may not sound that long, there may be times when it feels longer because it is so different from what your body is used to. Ask some of your friends and family, or even see there is a Facebook group of people who would like to do the cleanse with you.

You will add extra incentive to reach your goal when you have another person holding you accountable, or if there some fun competition added in. You don't have to be in the state, or even the same country to do this. As long as the two, or more, of you can stay in contact with each other, that's all that matters. Check in every few hours, or at least send a picture to one another of what you are eating.

Get Your Fridge Ready

Once you feel that you have sufficiently gotten your body and mind ready for your cleanse, you need to move onto your refrigerator. To ensure success, you will want to make sure that you have gotten rid of all of the temptations that you can by going through your fridge and cabinets.

The first thing you should do is make sure that your fridge is full of Dr. Sebi approved vegetables and fruits so that you will have what you need on hand for your fast. It's a good idea to have the fruits and veggies prepared in a way that makes it easy to just grab and use them. You can also go ahead and mix up your juices and smoothies that you will need for the week as well. You could also just have what you need for your juices and smoothies diced and in containers where all you have to do it throw it in the blender and go. When you have all of your food ready to go, it will save you some time in preparing your meals. It also means, if you start feeling hungry before you are suppose to eat next, you will have a quick snack that you can grab. This will lower the odds of you grabbing something not so healthy.

If you live with other people who won't be doing this cleanse with you, then you may not be able to throw out all of the bad foods. If they have snacks that don't have to be refrigerated, ask them to put them up somewhere so that you can't see them and don't know where they are. It may also be a good idea to keep your food separate from theirs in the fridge. This just ensures the things you need for the week don't get used up by accident.

You can prep any salads you may need for the week by fixing them in a mason jar. Make sure that the dressing is placed on the bottom and everything is stacked on top. Also, have a gallon of spring water drawn up at the end of each day ready for the next day. It is also a good idea to have a glass of water with you during the day. This can help with the hunger you might experience.

Be Easy With Yourself

We are all just human. We aren't perfect and messing up happens even if we have planned as much as we can. If you find that you end up given into temptation and mess up a bit, don't simply throw in the towel and give up. The cup of coffee or that piece of chocolate doesn't mean you're a failure, and does not mean you should stop your cleanse. A slip up may slow down your progress, but it does not bring it to a stop.

You are doing this cleanse for you and nobody else. If you slip, realize what happened, and then get back on track for your next meal. You may even notice that eating "off cleanse" makes you feel crappy. You may feel like your energy slumped, you develop of headache, or you may feel bloated. When this happens, simply recommit. Remind yourself of what your goal is and then remember that the next meal you have is another chance to make a different choice.

Lastly, I would like to suggest you compare yourself before and after. Before you start the cleanse take a picture of yourself from angles, measure your chest, waist, hips, upper arm, and thighs, and weight yourself. Also, write down how you have been feeling before the detox, such as tired, bloated, sluggish, and so on. During the detox, and this plays into your journaling, you can keep track of how you feel each day. Try to avoid re-measuring or weighing yourself during the detox. Then the morning of the first day off of the cleanse, so the eighth day, take new pictures, measurements, and weight. Then jot down how you are feeling. Do you have more energy? Do you feel motivated to eat healthier? Did you enjoy your experience? And so on.

Taking this step to do a cleanse is a big step, but I'm certain you can do it.

Chapter 1:The Dr. Sebi Treatment

The research of Western medicine has stated that diseases are caused by a person being infected by bacteria, viruses, or germs. To help a person overcome this "infestation," doctors provide them with inorganic chemicals. Dr. Sebi's research found the flaws in this premise through simple deductive reasoning. Western medicine has consistently used these same methods, and they have always provided people with the same ineffective results.

Instead, if we look at the African approach to diseases, it opposes Western medicine. The African Bio-mineral Balance rejects the bacteria, virus, and germ theory. Dr. Sebi's research found that diseases are able to grow when the mucous membrane is compromised. For example, if your bronchial tubes have too much mucus, the person is diagnosed with bronchitis. If the mucus is in the lungs, then they have pneumonia. When it moves to the pancreatic duct, they have diabetes. All of the compounds in the African Bio-mineral Balance are made up of natural plants, which make it alkaline.

This is very important in reversing these pathologies because diseases are only able to live in acidic environments. It doesn't make sense to use inorganic compounds to treat diseases because they are acidic. The consistent use of natural remedies will detoxify and cleanse a diseased body and will bring it back to its alkaline state.

Dr. Sebi's nutrition system takes things a step further. Besides getting rid of years of toxin build-up, the African Bio-mineral Balance will replace all of the depleted minerals and will rejuvenate any cell tissue that has been damaged by acid. The main organs that it helps are the colon, kidneys, lymph glands, gall bladder, liver, and skin. When the toxins are released from one of these organs, they will move through the body and manifest in disease. Eventually, the body will start to attack the weakest organ because it is unable to get rid of the toxin. The colon is probably one of the most important organs and needs to be cleansed before diseases are able to be reversed. But, if you only cleanse the colon, all of the other organs will still be toxic, which leaves the body diseased.

Through Dr. Sebi's intra-cellular detoxifying cleanse, every cell within the body will be purified. The body is then able to rejuvenate and rebuild itself.

Dr. Sebi's Diet

The Dr. Sebi diet is a plant-based alkaline diet. It helps to rejuvenate the cells in your body by getting rid of the toxic waste. The bulk of the diet is made up of a shortlist of foods along with supplements.

Dr. Sebi's diet is also able to help conditions like lupus, AIDS, kidney disease, and other diseases. The treatments for these diseases require you to eat only certain grains, fruits, and veggies, and strictly abstaining from animal products.

This is a very low protein diet, and that's what makes Dr. Sebi's supplements so important. You cannot have soy or animal products, lentils, or beans. You have several different options when it comes to Dr. Sebi's supplement choices, and you can even purchase and "all-inclusive" package that has 20 different products and can help to restore your body's health.

If you don't want to do the "all-inclusive" package, you can pick supplements according to the health problems you are suffering from. For example, Bio Ferro can help to increase overall wellbeing, help digestive issues, promote weight loss, boost immunity, cleanse the blood, and treat liver problems.

Weight Loss

While Dr. Sebi's diet isn't meant to be a weight loss diet, it can help you to lose weight. Since you will be cutting out all of the processed foods that most Western diets are made of, as well as fats, sugar, salt, and calories, you will likely lose weight.

Dr. Sebi's diet is a plant-based, vegan diet, and people who follow a plant-based diet often have a lower rate of heart disease and obesity. Plus, most of the foods you are allowed to eat are low in calories, except for oils, avocados, seeds, and nut, so even if you were to eat a lot of these foods, it is very unlikely that you are going to gain weight.

Benefits

Since you will be consuming a large number of fruits and veggies, it provides your body with many health benefits. Diets that are rich in fruits and veggies have been connected to less oxidative stress and reduced inflammation and can help to protect you from many different diseases.

Dr. Sebi's diet will also have you eating healthy fats and fiber-rich whole grains. All of these foods are connected to a lower risk of heart disease. Plus, you will be limiting those horrible processed foods, which is connected to better overall diet quality.

The biggest issue, though, that people have with Dr. Sebi's diet is that it is very restrictive and cuts out entire food groups that most people are used to eating. Plus, it can get very restrictive on the types of fruit and vegetables you are allowed to eat. Some people may struggle with this, but with some guidance and planning, you can make the switch.

Dr. Sebi Food List Recipes:

The Real 7-Day-Detox Method Cleanse with Approved Foods Following a Step-by-Step Dr. Sebi Alkaline Diet

M.S. Greger

Table of Contents

Introduction

First off, I would like to congratulate you for choosing *Dr. Sebi Food List Recipes* and taking a huge leap towards optimal health. Dr. Sebi was an amazing herbalist and naturalist, and has shown many people the best way to reach amazing health.

While there may be many people out there who don't understand Dr. Sebi, there are just as many who know that his teachings are helpful. If this is the first time you have ever heard of Dr. Sebi, let me take a moment to introduce you to him.

Dr. Sebi was born in Honduras as Alfredo Bowman. He was a self-taught man, and studied herbs all over the Americas and Africa. While he was taught about herbs from his grandmother at a young age, it was when he moved to America that he really dove into his studies.

Once in America, he was diagnosed with several diseases, but none of the remedies helped. That is when he went to an herbalist in Mexico. He saw great success with the herbalist, and this inspired his Dr. Sebi's Cell Food. Through the years he has helped many people, along with some celebrities.

This book is here to present to you Dr. Sebi's 7-day detox. This will help to reset your body and prepare it for a healthy future. Throughout the book, you will learn about Dr. Sebi's food list, his 10 commandments, and how to prepare yourself for the detox.

The great thing is, you can take the food list and continue to follow Dr. Sebi's diet after you have finished the detox. You will also feel amazing and your body will be thanking your for making it healthier.

Disclaimer

Please note that we are not doctors and we do not claim to be.
We simply follow the instructions of Dr. Sebi.

Chapter 1: Before You Begin

There are many different types of cleanses, from fasting to whole-foods, but they all aim to accomplish the same thing, and that is to get rid of inflammatory substances and toxicity. Then they provide your body with pure forms of nutrients. The goal of a cleanse is to heal and restore your body to its optimal health, and give its powerful detoxification systems to work without the blockages that are normally there.

The occasional detox is great for the body, but you should never just jump straight into a detox. Getting your body ready for the detox is just as important as the actual detox. If you already follow a very healthy and clean diet, then you won't have as much to do to get ready. But if you are like most people and follow a standard American diet, then you will have some work to do.

Cleanse and detox are words that tend to be used interchangeably, but they aren't quite the same thing. A cleanse is something that you do that will cause detoxification. Your body detoxes naturally as soon as your food has been digesting. This is where it will remove toxic and foreign materials. Unfortunately, the regular lifestyle and diets of most people causes them to accumulate more toxins than the body is able to purge. Because of this, we need to, on occasion, do a cleanse or fast where we consciously reduce the number of toxins that we are consuming so that the body is forced into a natural detoxifying state.

A cleanse could be a complete abstinence from food or toxic activities, and you only consume water. This type of fast might be helpful, but it's pretty hard to keep up. The Dr. Sebi detox won't require you to stop eating altogether, but if you want to try that type of cleanse, feel free to because it can do amazing things to your body.

Starting just a few days before you plan on beginning your detox, you will want to start changing how you eat. You will need to eat simple, light foods like salads, soups, or veggies. You will want to focus on raw veggies and leafy greens. This is especially true if you haven't been much of a clean eater. You need to give you body a chance to get ready for the cleanse. Take little steps by slowly cutting out processed and sugar foods, and star to increase you intake of fresh foods and grains.

Taking these small steps will increase your body's alkalinity to help it get ready for the deeper cleanse of your detox. During the detox, your body is going to end up releasing toxins that are stored in your tissues. These toxins may enter your bloodstream and can end up causing trouble sleeping, mood swings, body odor, bad breath, aches and pains, or rashes. By preparing for your detox, you can minimize your chances of developing these side effects.

To help you out, we will go over some tips on getting your body ready for your detox.

Dietary Changes

- Begin Your Day Right

You should start adding in a glass of warm lime water to your daily routine. This helps to jump-start your digestion and boost your metabolism. Lime juice is very alkalizing to your body, rich in vitamin C, and helps to cleanse your liver, which are all very important parts of detoxification.

- Switch Up Your Drinks

You will want to start drinking more spring water during the day, and start adding in some cleansing herbal teas, such as burdock, dandelion root, or nettle tea. This is also the best time to switch from regular tap water to spring water. You have to drink spring water while on Dr. Sebi's detox.

If you drink alcohol or coffee, you need to start cutting back on your consumption of them. You won't be able to have them on the detox. To let go of coffee, a good alternative is herbal or green tea. While green tea does contain caffeine, it is full of antioxidants, which will help your detoxification. Sodas and energy drinks should also be eliminated.

Water will play a very big part in your life, so beginning your day with two glasses of water is helpful in getting ready for your detox. If you choose to do the hot lime water, that counts towards a glass.

- Keep Things Simple

Start to change you meals to something that is very simple and easy to make. You should opt for dishes that are heavy in natural fruits and vegetables and start weaning yourself off of meats, if you are a meat eater. Include a lot of foods that are rich in chlorophyll because these aid in detoxification.

This can also include drinking veggie soups and broths. If you find it hard to eat enough vegetables, you can get your veggie intake through smoothies or juice. An easy way to add more fruits and veggies into your current diet is by adding a piece of organic fresh fruit to your breakfast each morning. You can also turn to fresh fruits as your mid-afternoon snack instead of heading to the vending machine. When picking out your fruits and veggies, go with organic, seasonal, and local produce when you can so that you avoid pesticides.

- Reduce Your Animal Product Intake

You are going to have to cut out animal products completely on Dr. Sebi's fast, so leading up to it, you should start weaning yourself off of them. The first place to start is to stop eating processed and red meats. This includes things like cured meats and sausages. Choosing leaner meats and fish is a better choice during this time. When picking fish, stay away from fish that are high in mercury, like mackerel and tuna. Fish like salmon, scallops, anchovies, and shrimp are better options.

- Check Your Oils

A lot of people will cook with vegetable or canola oil because the health industry tells you they are better because they are lower in fat, but they aren't. You need to start using olive oil, avocado oil, coconut oil, and grapeseed oil. Coconut and olive oils should not be cooked and should only be used raw. You can also use these oils along with some lime juice and herbs to create your own salad dressings.

- Up Your Grain Intake

Right now, you don't have to worry about eating Dr. Sebi approved grains. All you need to worry about is increasing how much whole grains you eat. Start eating more brown rice or spelt, and also start eating more pseudo-grains like quinoa. You need to start reducing how much refined foods like pasta and bread you consume, and that includes whole-grain bread or pasta. Do your best to avoid wheat wherever you are able to.

- Get Rid of Refined Sugar

You have to start reading nutrition levels to make sure that foods aren't hiding sugars. Before the detox, you can pick healthier sugar alternatives in moderation. Maple syrup, raw honey, rapadura sugar, coconut blossom syrup, coconut sugar, or agave nectar are great alternatives. Once the detox starts, you will only be able to have agave nectar.

- Get Rid of Table Salt

Table salt does not provide you with any nutrients. Your body also has a very hard time metabolizing table salt. While you are checking nutrition labels for sugars, check and make sure they aren't hiding any table salts. The majority of processed foods will have large amounts of chemically processed salts. You should use sea salt as your salt source. It is full of minerals and they are able to help get rid of heavy metals within your body.

- Cut Out Unhealthy Foods

Leading up to the detox, you should slowly start cutting out unhealthy foods that you like to eat. This includes things like store-bought cookies or muffins, chips, and fried foods. Choose, instead, to snack on homemade dried fruit, seeds, and unsalted nuts. Before the detox, feel free to try some raw chocolate to help you with your chocolate fix.

Get Your Mind Ready

But what should we do about the mind? There is a lot of evidence that has found that our mental state, from stressed to relaxed and all that is in between, has a large impact on our wellbeing and health. While you can do a cleanse for a week without changing anything else about your day, and you may feel pretty good after, but, when you add mindfulness into your cleanse, you will uncovering some amazing opportunities to move your focus inwards to create as much space in your emotional body and mind as you can in the physical body.

You could possibly be at a time of transition and you're looking for a fresh start to push yourself into the next phase. You could be holding onto something, such as a loss, fear, resentment, or unhealthy relationship, that you want to get rid of. Maybe most of your day is spent focusing on and caring for other people and feel like you need to do something for yourself. A lot of use resist turning in, and may even fear it. You could have an inner voice asking you to stop distracting yourself in order to listen to your intuition.

In order to get the most from your cleanse, it is a good idea to like what you want to get rid of other than the junk in your diet, and why you are drawn to this cleanse.

- Relax And Meditate

Getting ready for the cleanse doesn't just mean getting your belly ready for the change in foods, but it also means making sure your mind is ready for the change. Relaxation and mediation are a big part of detoxing because they can help you to reduce or eliminate your stress. Stress is the number one cause of so many unhealthy habits, such snacking on junk food or overeating. If you simply set aside some time each day to simple sit and be still, it will help to quiet your mind. This will help you to remain focused on what your goals are.

- Start Journalling

It's also a good idea to start keeping a detox journal. While you are getting ready for your detox, you can take the time to write out the guidelines for it, or simply write out what you hope it will do for you. In it, you should also make sure you schedule rest time. Your body will be doing a lot of work, and it's common to start feeling tired. Making sure you have rest time set aside will help to combat any fatigue you may experience. While detoxing, you can expel mental toxins by writing in the journal. You can write anything you want so that you mentally cleanse yourself. Let the words flow and don't worry if it makes sense, is grammatically correct, or what have you. Simply writing things out on paper is very therapeutic.

- Clear Your Space

While this might not seem important, but before you start cleaning your insides, you should also clean your outside. It has been proven that the health of mind is greatly impacted by your surroundings and all of the environmental toxins lurking in your space. Take the time to vacuum the floor, give your sheets a change, and use an air filter. You should also create your own sanctuary that you can use during your cleanse. This could be an entire room in your house, if you have a spare one, or it could simply be a comfy chair placed next to a window. Wherever you place your sanctuary, remove all of the clutter and place a vase of some of your favorite flowers or simply a photo that makes you happy. You can also choose something that calms or inspires you.

- Let Your Family and Friends Know

You are getting ready to embark on something that is likely going to be very different from your everyday life. That means, anybody you socialize with on a regular basis is probably going to notice something. Those that you live with will definitely notice something. To make sure that you are successful at your cleanse you will want to let your inner circle know what you are doing. Make sure that you get everybody on the same page so that they will know why you can't do certain things or go out to certain places during your weeklong cleanse. Your closest friends and family tend to be your biggest cheerleaders, so they may just be the person you turn to when you feel like giving up.

That being said, don't be surprised if you one of them question you about your choice of cleanse. If this happens, simply explain to them why you want to do this. If that's not good enough for them, don't try to change their mind. You don't have to have their approval to do this. You are doing this only for you, and not for them. If you have to keep your distance from them during the cleanse, then do so. Do what is best for you.

- Change Up Your Inner Dialogue

You know all of the negativity that tends to be swarming around in your head? You know that defeatist inner monologue that everybody tends to slip into from time to time? Now, is all of that serving you at all? When you start telling yourself that you aren't good enough, smart enough, skinny enough, and so, does it help you reach your goals? It is now time for you to change that inner dialogue. What though patterns will you be able to let go of as you are cleansing? To help you out, try writing down the negative things that you have told yourself. Underneath that negative thought, in bigger letters, change that negative sentence into a positive one. Things like "I can do anything I set

9

my mind to," "I am worthy," or "I am beautiful the way I am" are all great choices. You should also think about making this your mantra for your cleanse. You should say this out loud each and every day. At first, you might not believe the words coming out of your mouth, but after awhile, you will start to believe it.

- Pick a Good Time

While there likely is no perfect time to do a detox, it's a good idea to look at your calendar to see when you have the most free time. If you do, by chance, of a week of vacation built up at work and haven't made any other plans that might be a good option that way you don't have to worry about work. It's also a good idea to make sure that you detox won't occur during any major life events, holidays, important projects at work, or vacations. You definitely don't want to have a marathon run scheduled during the time you plan on doing your detox. It is just for a week, so it shouldn't be too hard to find at least one week where you don't have a lot going on.

- Think About a Digital Detox

This isn't something that you have to do, but it might be a good option if you are able to. Try to go digital-free for at least one whole day during your cleanse. The majority of people carry incredible power around with us in the form of tiny computers in your pocket. Remember, this cleanse that you have planned is time that you have set aside for yourself in order to remove junk from your life and replenish you system with healthy things.

This is true for your mind just as much as it is for your entire body. When you are going to the gym or heading out somewhere, leave your phone at home. Switch off your social media notifications. Choose one or two hours during the day to go through your emails or create an away message to let people know that you will get back to them tomorrow. Now that you have carved out some undistracted time, do something fun or healthy, like reading a book, write a letter, take a walk, or work on that project you have been meaning to for months. Whatever you want to do, that doesn't have to do with the digital world, do it.

- Lean Into Your Breath

When you start to experience the emotional or physical side effects of the cleanse, take a few minutes to simply breath so that you can connect with your body. This will help to slow your heart rate, help you to deal with imagined or real hunger, push through your erratic energy or mood swing, and then move the focus on your mind back into focus.

To do this, all you need to do is either stand or sit still and let your eyes close gently, or leave them open if you need to. Then take ten deep breaths in through your nose and release them out your mouth. As you inhale, picture it as a cleansing energy and view your exhale as a release of negativity. This can easily be done anywhere, like sitting in traffic or at the grocery store. Simply moving your attention to the movement of your breath will help to bring you into the present moment.

- Find a Cleanse Buddy

This might not be possible, but see if you can create some support for yourself and find somebody to do the cleanse with you. While a week may not sound that long, there may be times when it feels longer because it is so different from what your body is used to. Ask some of your friends and family, or even see there is a Facebook group of people who would like to do the cleanse with you.

You will add extra incentive to reach your goal when you have another person holding you accountable, or if there some fun competition added in. You don't have to be in the state, or even the same country to do this. As long as the two, or more, of you can stay in contact with each other, that's all that matters. Check in every few hours, or at least send a picture to one another of what you are eating.

Get Your Fridge Ready

Once you feel that you have sufficiently gotten your body and mind ready for your cleanse, you need to move onto your refrigerator. To ensure success, you will want to make sure that you have gotten rid of all of the temptations that you can by going through your fridge and cabinets.

The first thing you should do is make sure that your fridge is full of Dr. Sebi approved vegetables and fruits so that you will have what you need on hand for your fast. It's a good idea to have the fruits and veggies prepared in a way that makes it easy to just grab and use them. You can also go ahead and mix up your juices and smoothies that you will need for the week as well. You could also just have what you need for your juices and smoothies diced and in containers where all you have to do it throw it in the blender and go. When you have all of your food ready to go, it will save you some time in preparing your meals. It also means, if you start feeling hungry before you are suppose to eat next, you will have a quick snack that you can grab. This will lower the odds of you grabbing something not so healthy.

If you live with other people who won't be doing this cleanse with you, then you may not be able to throw out all of the bad foods. If they have snacks that don't have to be refrigerated, ask them to put them up somewhere so that you can't see them and don't know where they are. It may also be a good idea to keep your food separate from theirs in the fridge. This just ensures the things you need for the week don't get used up by accident.

You can prep any salads you may need for the week by fixing them in a mason jar. Make sure that the dressing is placed on the bottom and everything is stacked on top. Also, have a gallon of spring water drawn up at the end of each day ready for the next day. It is also a good idea to have a glass of water with you during the day. This can help with the hunger you might experience.

Be Easy With Yourself

We are all just human. We aren't perfect and messing up happens even if we have planned as much as we can. If you find that you end up given into temptation and mess up a bit, don't simply throw in the towel and give up. The cup of coffee or that piece of chocolate doesn't mean you're a failure, and does not mean you should stop your cleanse. A slip up may slow down your progress, but it does not bring it to a stop.

You are doing this cleanse for you and nobody else. If you slip, realize what happened, and then get back on track for your next meal. You may even notice that eating "off cleanse" makes you feel crappy. You may feel like your energy slumped, you develop of headache, or you may feel bloated. When this happens, simply recommit. Remind yourself of what your goal is and then remember that the next meal you have is another chance to make a different choice.

Lastly, I would like to suggest you compare yourself before and after. Before you start the cleanse take a picture of yourself from angles, measure your chest, waist, hips, upper arm, and thighs, and weight yourself. Also, write down how you have been feeling before the detox, such as tired, bloated, sluggish, and so on. During the detox, and this plays into your journaling, you can keep track of how you feel each day. Try to avoid re-measuring or weighing yourself during the detox. Then the morning of the first day off of the cleanse, so the eighth day, take new pictures, measurements, and weight. Then jot down how you are feeling. Do you have more energy? Do you feel motivated to eat healthier? Did you enjoy your experience? And so on.

Taking this step to do a cleanse is a big step, but I'm certain you can do it.

Chapter 2: What to Expect From the Detox

Some people go into a detox without knowing exactly what to expect. Dr. Sebi's detox plan will help clean out your system while freeing your system of stress and getting rid of all the toxins in your system.

There are four main causes of most diseases and they are:

- The body has too many toxins

- The body has a deficiency in nutrients

- The body's electromagnetic system is in chaos

- There is too much stress in the body

You might not understand these steps but you will soon realize that these problems are huge. While our bodies get older, they are getting more and more toxic. Most Americans today are addicted to fast food. It is just too easy to drive through a fast food restaurant and grab a burger and fries before going home. It is too easy to put a frozen dinner in the oven or microwave rather than making a huge salad or making some smoothies. All diseases begin in our stomachs.

The Body Has Too Many Toxins

There is only one way to get all the toxins out of our bodies and that is to fast and cleanse. When we don't eat, we are starving all the parasites that are living in our bodies. This allows all the bad things to leave our bodies through our feces and urine. Most people don't like to think about parasites living in their bodies but unfortunately we all do.

We have to eat a strict diet full of fruit and vegetables along with fasting. Stay away from grains at this point. Anyone who has followed Dr. Sebi's for any time know that cleansing is an essential part of the system.

During this time, you have to concentrate on everything that goes into your body:

- Make sure you drink a whole gallon of spring water each day

- Stop eating by 6 pm

- Cook your meals at home

- Never eat any prepackaged shakes or foods

- Use only date sugar, date syrup, or agave syrup as sweeteners

- Get a good juicer so you are able to make your own juice

- Eat one organic apple each day

- Consume as many herbal teas as you would like

- Take the Bromide Mix plus the Green Food Plus Daily

- Season using sea salt

- Consume organic, raw seeds and nuts

- Never consume anything that has been labeled as fat free or diet

- Never drink diet sodas

- Never consume any sweetener other than the above

- Never consume anything that has been stored in plastic

- Never consume anything that is cooked in a microwave

- Buy organic foods if you can afford them
- Never eat fast foods
- Never drink water from your tap
- Only consume the oils that have been approved by Dr. Sebi
- Don't eat grains during this cleanse
- Never eat packaged foods like pasta
- Consume all the vegetables and fruits that have been approved by Dr. Sebi
- Find deodorants, anti-perspirants, and sunblock that are chemical free
- Use an essential oil diffuser and pick three oils that will help you sleep
- Jump on a mini trampoline for 30 minutes a day
- Make sure your cleaning supplies are all natural
- Practice some deep breathing
- Do yoga or pilates to stretch your muscles
- Walk one hour each day
- Don't use steam rooms, swimming pools or hot tubs
- Get rid of all florescent lighting
- Don't use air fresheners
- Limit how long you use an air conditioner
- Don't dry clean your clothes

- Get a good vacuum cleaner that has a hepa filter

- Don't take OTC vitamins except vitamin D3 and digestive enzymes

- Go outside daily and enjoy the sun

- Make sure your toothpaste doesn't have fluoride

Cut Back on Using Electromagnetic Devices

- Lower your television time.

- Cut back on the amount of time you use wireless and electromagnetic devices.

- If at all possible get a mattress pad that is magnetic.

- Find rings that are magnetic.

- Sleep with a magnetic eye mask.

- Don't use electric tumble dryers

- Place some potted plants in your house.

- Wear white

- Try to Feng Shui your office and home.

Getting Rid of Stress

- Plant a garden

- Find your purpose in life

- Write down your goals

- If you aren't allergic, adopt a pet

- Try TFT. Tapping can reduce fears, anxiety, and stress.

- Foot orthodics

- Be thankful each day

- Listen to music you love

- Be kind recklessly

- Have sex

- Don't watch the news or read the papers

- Take a 15 minute break each afternoon

- Try to go to be no later than 10 pm

- Get up eat day by 6pm

- Rest from Friday evening until Saturday evening

- Try to sleep for at least eight hours

- Never use your cell phone while driving

- Use powerful words when you talk

- Give hugs

- Smile

- Try to listen to CDs that reduce stress.

- Laugh more

Doctor Sebi's Diet

This diet works based on this two fold approach:

1. Cleanses our bodies of toxins and waste by fasting

2. Nourishing our bodies on a cellular level by eating foods that are alkalizing and free of starch

After your body has been cleansed of as many toxins and waste that has been created over time, it will then be able to take in everything it needs to take its healing power up a notch.

Dr. Sebi believes that if our bodies are acidic, it was being exposed to more diseases. Because of this, his diet was created to bring alkalizing foods into our bodies to help flush out all the toxins and bring in the minerals that have been depleted.

All the damaged tissues that acidity had messed up could recover and be rejuvenated by eating certain foods. You will soon be able to see better health in your colon, gall bladder, lymph glands, liver, kidneys, and skin.

This diet takes on a holistic approach to treat the whole person rather than just a symptom or two. This is called intercellular cleansing. This diet cured Dr. Sebi of many problems that common doctors weren't able to.

What Will Happen During Detox

The first step when overcoming addiction to anything is dealing with our body's dependency on foods and sugar. When you finally make the decision to detox your body is an act of courage. You are actually admitting that you need help and are ready to get healthy.

You need to know what can happen during this part of your journey. Detoxing can be stressful and painful. It is going to take a lot of dedication and hard work.

In this day and age, our bodies are being assaulted constantly by different toxins. We ingest these toxins through what we drink and eat. Toxins in the environment attack us daily. Toxins also get created because of things inside our bodies.

The liver tries to clean all these toxins but eventually its ability to efficiently detoxify gets inhibited because of being constantly loaded down by more toxins that it can filter out.

Once the body can't get rid of these toxins any more, they get stored as fat and we have to deal with it later. If we don't give our bodies a chance to get these toxins out of our bodies, they are going to build up and create a condition known as fatty liver.

When we detox, we are minimizing the toxins that our bodies have to process. We are giving our livers what it needs to begin processing toxins once more. When they have been processed, they get released into the blood, kidneys, and lymphatic system to get eliminated. Leaving too many toxins in our bodies can cause a lot of health concerns and problems.

Let's look at some benefits of detoxing, foods that will help the body detox, and what will happen to our bodies that will cause a "healing crisis," or "detoxing effect."

Why Detox?

- Reduces your dependency on things such as refined carbs, caffeine, and sugars.

- Reduced increased body fats, acne, inflammation, aches, headaches, among other things.

- Gets rid of environmental toxins that have been building up in your body.

- Helps to repair damage and rebalance the body.

What is Happening in Your Body While Detoxing

- The Explanation

Everyone will begin detoxing for various reasons and everyone is going to have a different level of toxicity. When trying to give a simple explanation, it is important to remember that everyone's body is unique to them. Because of this, everybody will have a different experience when they are detoxing and will have various symptoms.

One rule to remember is the more toxic a body is, or if they have more years of bad eating habits, the more intense the healing crisis is going to be.

When you begin a detox, you might notice some symptoms get a whole lot worse. This is completely normal and happens when our bodies begin clearing out all the built up sludge. This is completely natural and just a process of the body healing itself by getting rid of all the toxins that have built up in your cells.

This is normally called the "detox reaction." We think of it as a "healing reaction" or a "healing crisis." It is a necessary evil where you are going to feel worse for a few days before you begin to feel any better.

All the bad toxins get expelled from your body in this process. These toxins might have been trapped in your cells, gallbladder, or liver for years and possibly decades. The more toxic your body is or if you have had bad habits for a long time, your healing crisis is going to be more intense. The organs that get rid of these toxins like the kidneys, liver, skin, and lungs work together to get rid of all these waste products but it can be an overwhelming process.

You need to remember that what you are going through will only be temporary and you are walking a path of renewed health. Although this time is very uncomfortable, it's a good sign that your body is doing what it needs to do to heal itself. This normally lasts about two to five days.

- Sugar Detox

If you have tried to reduce the amount of sugar that you eat, you probably became extremely aware of just how hard it is to stop eating sugar. This is called "sugar withdrawals." This is the body's way of getting rid of its dependency on using sugar to make energy.

During this process, there are some things that are being changed and now your body need to do more to break down fats in order to make energy. This is similar to the way a muscle has to be trained. But with time it gets stronger and is able to do things better and faster. In the beginning, you will experience some detoxing symptoms and you might feel more tired.

Plus, if you eat sugar, your body is going to use all the insulin that it makes when you eat sugar to create neurotransmitters that make you feel good. When you reduce the amount of sugar you eat, your body will work a lot harder to make those neurotransmitters. This could cause you to experience strong emotional swings and headaches while your body gets adjusted.

- Alcohol Detox

Alcohol is basically sugar. You won't experience any side effects from detoxing off sugar unless you are an alcoholic and your body has become dependent on it. The only effect you are going to experience would be the neurotransmitters that we talked about above.

- Caffeine Detox

The effect that caffeine has on our bodies and brains is extremely complicated. When you drink caffeine, it constricts the blood vessels in your brain and reduces the blood flow. If you reduce the amount of caffeine you get each day, you will be increasing the amount of blood that flows to the brain and this can make pain receptors become more sensitive and this in turn creates the "caffeine headache."

- Helping Your Body Detox
  - o Make sure your body has all the daily nutrients that your body needs to help your organs get rid of the toxins

- You need to make sure you have a good bowel movement each day. This makes sure your body is getting rid of the toxins and keeps them from getting absorbed back into your body.

- Exfoliate and dry brush

- Don't do any intense workouts. Do some lighter stuff like yoga or walking that gets your blood flowing without adding more stress of the body.

- Let your body rest and get lots of sleep

- Drink more water

You need to remember that all the symptoms you are experiencing during your "healing crisis" will just be temporary. You are walking a path to better health. Although these symptoms are uncomfortable, it's a good sign that your body is doing what it needs to do to heal itself. These symptoms normally last around two to five days.

Getting Rid of Toxins by Doing a Metabolic Detox

A metabolic detox is pretty much just like any other detox. It helps the body find and get rid of toxins. Our bodies are exposed to environmental and endogenous toxins daily. There are some cases that our bodies don't get rid of all the toxins and then they accumulate in our tissues and organs. This disrupts our normal cellular functions and increases our risk of getting diseases. Using a metabolic detox can support our body's system and helps to reduce the toxic burden on our bodies. This is crucial for our longevity and health.

- Types of Toxins

  - Bacterial endotoxins

  - Industrial chemicals

- o   Plastics

- o   Pesticides

- o   Heavy metals

- Detoxification Systems

One important component of a metabolic detox is to support all of our body's elimination pathways because toxins have to leave the body through sweat, urine, and stool. The phases of cellular detox needs to be supported, too. This type of support creates the basis of any successful metabolic detox plan.

- Common Symptoms and Solutions

Most people will experience some symptoms during their metabolic detox especially if it is their first detox. These symptoms might happen once the process gets unbalanced or the toxins aren't gotten rid of properly. This is a biological problem where the toxins that are released are more than the body's ability to transport them and then sufficiently eliminate them. These symptoms are normally minor and only last a few days.

1.   Irritability, Tiredness, and Headaches

These symptoms can develop rom suddenly stopping your intake of wheat, sugar, alcohol, and caffeine. All of these can be very addictive. Other things that can cause these symptoms are constipation, dehydrations, fluctuations in your blood sugar, and toxins not being released from all their hiding places.

Here are some possible solutions:

- o   Make sure your bowels are regular

- o   Get more and better sleep

- o Help stabilize your blood sugar by adding high quality oils and fiber for every meal.

- o Keep your body in an alkaline state by eating herbs, fruits, and vegetables.

- o Drink more water

2. Cravings

Most people will experience some cravings while doing any type of diet including a metabolic detox. Cravings will go away in a couple of days. There are some reasons why you might have some cravings during your detox:

- o Microbial imbalances in your digestive tract due to the change of diet

- o Breaking your sugar habits

- o Withdrawal from drinks and foods you might be addicted to

Because caffeine, gluten, and sugar can trigger a response in the brain similar to opioids and these foods can be very addictive. Sweets can trigger the release of serotonin which is the "feel good" neurotransmitters that creates an addiction to sugar.

The state of your microbiome could also affect some cravings. Certain strains will be associated with certain cravings. Your gut can trigger a craving that will favor a particular microbe, even though it could essential hurt you. These microbes could also cause you to feel bad until you feed that craving and then "euphoria" begins.

Metabolic detox and their components could help shift your microbiome and address specific aspects of dysbiosis, and help conquer your cravings for unhealthy foods is one reward you will get from all this.

Here are some solutions to help you through.

- o To avoid sugar cravings, drink smoothies and eat the right fruits.

- o Drink more alkaline beverages and foods in your diet. This can help minimize your food cravings and support the right shifts of your gut microbes.

For basic cravings, you can normally substitute other food that work within your diet.

3. Irregular Bowels

Constipation is the worst enemy of any detox plan. Most toxins in the body are sent out of the body through the bowels. Most meal plans that help the body detoxify normally include fiber-rich foods like vegetables. If you still have some digestive problems, you can try these solutions:

- o Physical activity can help improve regularity

- o High fiber seeds, vegetables that aren't starchy, along with healthy oils can help lubricate your digestive tract

- o Eat bitter herbs and vegetables

- o Drink herbal teas and water.

All of these can help you feel confident during your metabolic detox, even if your symptoms are very mild. Knowing why these symptoms happen and what you can do about them can help you reap all the benefits of your metabolic detox.

Chapter 3: Dr. Sebi Food List

Before we get into Dr. Sebi's list of foods, let's find out more about what alkalizing foods are and why we need them. Dr. Sebi's diet is essentially an alkaline diet that says it can improve your health, while helping you lose weight along with fighting off cancer cells.

An alkaline diet has the basis that there are certain foods that can cause our bodies to create acid which is very harmful to our bodies. It states that when we eat specific foods or drink specific beverages, you will be able to change your body's acid level. This is also known as your pH level. This scale measures how basic or acidic a food is based on a scale of 1 to 14. Foods that are alkaline will have a number that is greater than seven.

Some people think that if we can change our body's pH level, it will improve our health and can help us lose some weight.

The Conundrum about Acidity and Alkalinity

Some people wonder if the drinks and foods we consume daily could make our bodies and blood more acidic. This is very true. Since our bodies have a very complex nature, there is a lot more to it than just getting our bodies alkaline.

Since some parts of our bodies need to be acidic and others like our blood need to be alkaline and everything we eat along with life's stresses, what we drink, all affect that outcome. Let me try to explain it a bit better.

Our bodies are a complex set of various systems like the endocrine system, lymphatic system, digestive system, along with the eco system of muscles, bones, fats, fluids, organs, and nerves.

Some of these like the stomach need to be acidic just to be able to digest foods. Our stomachs are very acidic. Our blood stream should be a bit alkaline. Since the blood's plasma is vital to keeping the body's health systems functioning properly, the people who favor the alkaline diet are right. We should consume a diet that is alkaline to keep our bodies healthy.

If our diets are too acidic or when we eat too much grains, dairy, refined carbs, sugar, eggs, and meats, then our body's system begins breaking down and this will eventually make our blood too acidic. This is what all those experts left out when they said what we drink and eat doesn't affect our body's acidic and alkaline balance. It most certainly does. Sometimes it causes horrible consequences.

An acidic versus alkaline body could mean the difference between sickness and health, the difference between dying early of diabetes, cancer, or heart disease or living a long and healthy life. Let's find out more about how this happens.

The Hidden Truth about the Body's pH

Alkaline and acidity levels get measured by a pH scale of 1 to 14. Our stomachs have a pH level of one or two and this makes them very acidic. Blood, which has a pH level that is between 7.36 to 7.50 is slightly alkaline.

Our blood's pH level gets regulated by a system of buffers that work 24 / 7 to keep this narrow range of alkalinity. Because of this, most people who follow the paleo diet proclaim that you don't have anything to worry about. Just eat all the meat you want and you will be fine.

These paleo people tell us that our body's buffer system takes care of all this acidity. They claim that this is backed by science. If you look at your body's ecology, you will see that this idea isn't based on science. It is only a myth.

This means that the vegetarians, raw foodists, and vegans are correct. We have to eat alkaline foods to remain in optimal health. There are still most vegetarians and vegans who don't completely understand everything that is happening. Most vegetarians and vegans are too acidic and not in perfect health.

Although I have physically experienced some wonderful healthy changed by following Dr. Sebi's diet, it took me some time to understand the ecological science behind the improvements. The reasons lie in the subtlety and complexity of all the organs that are involved in absorption, digestion, and elimination of all the toxins in our bodies.

The True Story of the Advantages

The healthiest blood pH will be between 7.42 and 7.50. The cells can operate most efficiently at this range. Our health and life depends on our body's physiological power to keep the blood pH stable at about 7.46 through homeostasis.

This is the issue that people who deny how important alkaline foods are missing. It is the need to keep homeostasis. If you blood pH gets a bit less alkaline like below the range of 7.46 because of a breakdown in the buffer system of the body, then the body's mechanisms begin to break down, too.

How do we remain in homeostasis? We have to be sure that our body's buffering system doesn't get too overtaxed by consuming too many foods that are acidic. If the body gets too acidic, we might begin suffering from gall stones, kidney stones, osteoporosis, and other extremely undesirable health challenges.

Let's look at how fundamental pH is and how our bodies regulate the alkaline-acid balance of all its fluid every moment of every day.

Our body's pH keeps a measurement of how alkaline or acidic a liquid is. When talking about our physiology, the involved liquids are bodily fluids that can be put into two groups: the extracellular fluids like the plasma of blood and the interstitial fluids that fill the space around the tissues like the cardiovascular, nervous system, joints, lymphatic system, etc and the intracellular fluids that are found in our cells.

As stated above, our blood plasma has to maintain a pH level of around 7.46 in order to work right. Our cells require the three dimensional shapes to maintain homeostasis. The smallest of changes in the body's fluid pH will change the blood's pH, too. This is what most of the "experts" are leaving out.

Reading a pH Scale

Every number on the pH scale represents a difference that is tenfold from the number above or below it. This means that a liquid that has a pH of six is ten times more acidic that something that has a pH of seven. Something that has a pH of five is one hundred times more acidic than water.

Anytime we eat or drink anything, the end product of digestion and assimilation of the nutrients usually results in either an alkaline or acid-forming effect. These end products sometimes get called alkaline ash or acid ash.

Our cells also produce energy constantly. Various acids get formed and then released into the bodily fluids. These acids that are generated by our normal activities can't be avoided. If you body has to create energy to survive, it produces a constant acid supply.

There are two things that can disrupt our body's pH: the acids we generate by doing regular metabolic acitivites and the alkaline or acid-forming effects of liquids and foods.

Plus, stress could affect the acid levels in the body because we normally don't digest food properly if we are on the go constantly and are stressed. Fortunately, our bodies have three mechanisms to help prevent these things from shifting our blood's pH out of the optimal range.

Body's Buffer

Our bodies have a buffer system of carbonic acids, a phosphate buffer sstem, and a protein buffer system. Plus, we buffer ourselves when we exhale carbon dioxide and by getting rid of hydrogen through the kidneys.

It is because of these facts that experts say that certain foods can't have any negative effects on our health by effecting the acidity alkaline balance. Their main argument is our body's buffering system can take care of anything that we decide to eat.

This is so false it isn't even funny. When you eat junk food that contains too many refined carbs, sugars, and animal fats, the buffering system gets overloaded and can't protect the blood from getting too acidic. This means out bodies can maintain homeostasis. This is when we begin getting sick.

If our bodies are constantly exposed to huge quantities of liquids and foods that form acids, you body will call on its calcium phosphate reserves to give your phosphate buffer system what it needs to neutralize the acids in your diet. With time, this might lead to weaknesses in your teeth and bones.

Consuming a diet of acid-forming foods could increase the risk of developing kidney stones. One other common effect of a diet rich in acidic foods along with stress is acid-reflux. It is in your best interest not to overtax your body's buffering system by consuming foods that produce alkaline.

Alkaline Foods

All fruits and non-starchy vegetables will have an alkaline-forming effect of the body. This means that bananas and potatoes are a bit more acidic than other fruits and vegetables. Because of this, most non-starchy vegetables, berries, and fruits need to be the majority of your diet. Nature has made it so that leafy greens like bell peppers and kale are very alkaline. These are also some of the most nutrient foods that we can eat.

Refined grains and whole grains have an acidic effect of the body. Legumes are semi-alkaline. All sugar, dairy, fish, eggs, and every meat product are very acidic when they are digested. This means all these foods have to be eliminated from your diet.

Most animal foods, highly processed foods, and animal foods have an acid forming effect on the body. The best way to help you body is to consume a diet of alkaline forming foods.

Basically, if you are a vegan and live off of protein bars you will end up with an unhealthy and acidic blood stream. While an omnivore who eats a lot of vegetables and fruits can remain healthy and alkaline.

Basically, our bodies need to stay in homeostasis with a blood pH level or around 7.46 to keep us in good health. We can do this by eating a diet of alkaline producing foods that are made up of vegetables and fruits. These are also the most nutrient dense foods, too.

There isn't any need for vegans and paleo people to go to war regarding what is right or wrong with an alkaline diet. These facts speak for themselves. Basically, you can be acidic on any diet if you consume to many acid forming foods like refined carbs, sugar, fats, and animal protein along with too many foods that are deep fried. Whether to be an omnivore, vegetarian, or vegan is more of a question about ethics as long as what you eat is alkaline.

If you want to get and remain healthy, animal products and junk foods have to be eliminated and the majority of what you eat has to be alkaline.

Dr. Sebi's Food List

- Vegetables

As with all his foods, Dr. Sebi had a belief that we need to only eat foods that are non-GMO. This includes vegetables and fruits that have been altered to contain more minerals and vitamins or made seedless. This list of vegetables is diverse and rather large. There are lots of options so you can create a variety of meals.

o Zucchini

o Wild arugula

o Watercress

o Wakame

o Turnip greens

o Tomatillo

o Squash

o Purslane verdolaga

o Onions

o Olives

o Okra

o Nori

o Nopales

o Mushrooms except Shitake

o Lettuce except iceberg

o Kale

o Izote leaf and flower

o Hijiki

o Garbanzo beans

o Dulse

- o Dandelion greens
- o Cucumber
- o Plum and cherry tomato
- o Chayote
- o Bell pepper
- o Avocado
- o Arame
- o Amaranth

- Fruits

Even though the vegetable list is fairly long, the fruits are more restricted. Most of the fruits you would normally eat have been eliminated. The fruits that you are allowed to eat offer you some options. Every variety of berries are allowed with the exception of cranberries. These fruits are made by man.

- o Tamarind
- o Soursops
- o Soft jelly coconuts
- o Raisins
- o Prunes
- o Prickly pear
- o Plums
- o Pears
- o Peaches
- o Papayas

- o Orange

- o Melons

- o Mango

- o Limes

- o Grapes

- o Figs

- o Dates

- o Currants

- o Cherries

- o Cantaloupe

- o Berries

- o Bananas

- o Apples

- Herbs

This is the most limited list of all Dr. Sebi's foods because it is hard to find an herb that hasn't been altered. A good rule to remember is to think about the ones that can be used when they are harvested out of the garden. The most versatile herbs are:

- o Pure sea salt

- o Onion powder

- o Oregano

- o Dill

- o Cayenne

- Basil
- Herbal Teas
  - Tila
  - Red Raspberry
  - Ginger
  - Fennel
  - Elderberry
  - Chamomile
  - Burdock
- Sweeteners and sugars
  - 100 percent pure agave syrup
  - Date sugar
- Grains
  - Wild rice
  - Tef
  - Spelt
  - Rye
  - Quinoa
  - Kamut
  - Fonio
  - Amaranth
- Seasonings and Spices

- o Thyme
- o Tarragon
- o Sweet basil
- o Savory
- o Sage
- o Pure sea salt
- o Powdered granulated seaweed
- o Oregano
- o Onion powder
- o Habanero
- o Dill
- o Cloves
- o Cayenne
- o Bay leaf
- o Basil
- o Achiote

There are many dieters who thing that Dr. Sebi's food list is too limiting. His faithful followers feel that there is plenty of food to give them a variety. A normal meal with this diet could look something like a large green salad with olive oil dressing or veggies sautéed in avocado oil. Even though it might take some time to get used to, this list can be easy to follow and beneficial to your health.

Chapter 4: The 10 Commandments of Dr. Sebi

Dr. Sebi, on his nutritional guide, ends with eight rules to follow when on his diet. Those are fairly simple and straightforward, but here I am going to share the 10 commandments of Dr. Sebi when it comes to following this 7-day detox diet. These may overlap a bit with his nutritional guide rules. These commandments are rules that you should make sure that you follow to the best of your abilities while on the cleanse.

1. Do not eat processed foods while on the cleanse.

The point of a detox is to clean up your diet and to rid your body of junk that is in processed foods. This means you need to eat only the organic fruits, veggies, and grains that was in the food list above and will be in the recipes below. You also need to avoid all forms of sugar when on this detox.

2. Drink at least a gallon of spring water every day.

This is a requirement for the detox as well as the Dr. Sebi diet. Drinking lots of water will help to flush out the toxins in your body. If you haven't been drinking enough water, your urine will be dark in color. You want your urine to be a pale yellow. You also need to make sure that you buy spring water. Tap water is full of the added chemicals due to the processing it has to go through before it gets to you. Spring water is naturally alkaline and contains minerals that are beneficial to you. Do not choose distilled or purified water. These are not alkaline, and they will rob you of minerals that you need.

3. Stay away from unnatural detox pills.

A lot of people will purchase expensive pills that act as diuretics or laxatives to "help" them during their detox. You should not do this. They are not helping you, and they can become dangerous. These pills will cause you to lose essential electrolytes. And, they only make you lose water weight and nothing more.

4. Eliminate all alcohol and caffeine from your diet.

While you are detoxing you must eliminate all alcohol and caffeine from your body. These are toxins, and you want to eliminate toxins, right? Caffeine is a stimulant that will end up fatiguing your adrenal glands, and after awhile, they are going to end up making your more tired. Alcohol is a depressant and will hurt your liver. Instead, you should choose herbal teas that will help your liver and kidney function.

5. Eliminate all sources of animal products and hybrid foods.

The Dr. Sebi's diet is a vegan diet, and so is the detox. It has been known for a long time that animal products aren't that great for you, especially red meats. For example, dairy products are really hard for your body to digest. They are also high in saturated fats, which can raise your cholesterol. Hybrid foods are eliminated because they are not naturally found in nature. Hybrid foods are natural fruits and veggies that have been changed in the lab so that they grow bigger fruit.

6. Do not use the microwave for cooking your foods.

Microwave ovens release radiation and basically kill the nutrients in your foods. The radiation is also able to heat body tissue just like it heats your food. Any vitamin B 12 your food may have had in it is gone when it is heated in the microwave. It is also able to add carcinogens to your food and change your heart rate.

7. Do not use canned or pre-frozen fruits and veggies.

While canned or pre-frozen fruits and veggies may be a convenience, they do not have the same nutrients as fresh fruit and veggies that you prepare yourself. The cans contain BPA, bisphenoal-A, which is a chemical that can end up leeching into the food. Research has shown that eating canned food can end up leading to BPA exposure. BPA has been linked to health issues like male sexual dysfunction, type 2 diabetes, and heart disease. Plus, while it is extremely rare, canned foods can contain clostridium botulinum. If ingested, it can cause botulism, which is a serious illness that can end up causing paralysis and death.

8. Avoid any fruits that are made seedless.

Seedless fruits are created through a process known as parthenocarpy. This is a process of producing fruit with no fertilization. This can happen naturally through mutation or it can be created artificially, which can include synthetic chemicals. This process of producing seedless fruit removes some of the fiber content, and it can cause you to be exposed to chemicals if the fruit was made in a lab.

9. If taking, make sure you Dr. Sebi's products are taken an hour before pharmaceuticals.

Dr. Sebi offers supplements that you can take during your detox, and for the rest of your life if you want. This detox does not call for any of them explicitly, but you can check them out on his website and find out which you would like to take. He has complete packages of supplements specifically made for men and for women. If you don't want to start taking do many, you can simple choose to take the bromide plus powder and Bio Ferra. No matter what you choose to take, if you also take prescription drugs, you must take the supplements an hour before. This gives the supplements a chance to protect your body.

10. Stick to the grains in the food list and avoid wheat.

In 1 in 133 people gluten causes an autoimmune response that will attack your small intestine. That is a very common statistic.

Even if a person isn't that 1 in 133 with celiac disease, there are still a considerable number of people who are gluten intolerant. Even people who don't have a problem with gluten can experience gut inflammation from eating wheat. This is a completely different problem from gluten, and can end up causing problems for your health. Inflammation in your gut can end up leading to leaky gut syndrome. This isn't the kind of thing you want happening when you are trying to clean up your diet through your detox.

If you make sure you follow these 10 commandments, you will definitely see success in your detox.

Chapter 5: Detox Day One

We've made to the first day of the detox. This is what you have been waiting for, and, hopefully, excited about. On each day of the detox, you will find three recipes, two snacks, and a step-by-step guide to the day. This guide is only a suggestion, and you do not have to follow it to the T. For some people, following the guideline makes things easier so they are more likely to stick to the detox. If at any point during the day water does not help your hunger or you start to feel "off" you can eat a snack of any Dr. Sebi approved food. I would suggest bell pepper slices with homemade hummus or some olives.

Each day, start off your day with a glass of warm lime water. This will help to free your body of toxins.

Breakfast: Power Smoothie

What You Will Need:

Hemp seeds, .5 c

An apple

Grated ginger, .5 tsp

Water, 2 c

Amaranth greens, 1 c

Dandelion greens, 1 c

What You Will Do:

Start by cleaning the apple and greens. Core, peel, and chop the apple. Before grating the ginger, make sure that you remove the skin. Once you have your fruit and veggies ready, add them into your blender along with all of the other ingredients except for the water. Start blending everything together and slowly add the water in until it reaches you desired consistency. Enjoy.

Snack 1: Kale Chips

What You Will Need:

Sea salt

Grapeseed oil

Bundle of dinosaur kale

What You Will Do:

Start by ripping the kale leaves off of their stem. Rip them into smaller chip-sized pieces and then place them into a bowl. Add in some oil and salt and toss them altogether.

Spread the kale over a baking sheet. Make sure that you have your oven at 350. Bake your kale chips for 15 minutes. Enjoy

Lunch: Mixed Green Salad with Bell Pepper Dressing and Quinoa

What You Will Need:

Salad:

An avocado

Chopped red bell pepper, 1 c

Chopped cucumber

A large tomato

Your favorite Dr. Sebi approved mixed greens

Red Bell Pepper Dressing:

Water

Olive oil .5 c

Sea salt, 1.5 tsp

Lime juice, 3 tbsp

Dill, 2 tsp

Ginger, 1.5 tbsp

Chopped red bell pepper 1.75 c

Quinoa:

Boiling water, 1.5 to 1.75 c

Quinoa, 1 c

What You Will Do:

Start by cooking your quinoa since it will take the longest to prepare. Once your water is boiling, add in the quinoa and lower the heat and let it simmer for 20 minutes without being covered. The quinoa should be tender. If you find that the quinoa is still not fully cooked and the water has dried up, add in some extra water. If you want, you can mix in some sea salt and cayenne pepper.

As the quinoa cooks, you can prepare the dressing for your salad. Once you have prepped all of the ingredients, add everything to your blender and mix it altogether until it is well mixed. If the dressing looks too thick, drizzle in some water until it reaches a dressing-like consistency. Keep the dressing stored in a glass jar. It will keep in the fridge for 10 days. Give it a shake before using.

Once the dressing and quinoa is ready, you can put your salad together. All you need to do is toss the salad ingredients together. You can substitute any of the ingredients you want for any other veggie on the food list. You can also add in some garbanzo beans if you want to.

Drizzle your salad in two tablespoons of the dressing and serve the salad over the quinoa and enjoy.

Snack 2: Veggies and Guacamole

What You Will Need:

Lime juice, 3 tsp

Sea salt, .5 tsp

Onion powder, 2 tsp

Avocado, 2

Sliced bell pepper

Sliced cucumber

What You Will Do:

Mash the avocados together and then mix in the lime juice, salt, and onion powder. Enjoy the veggies in the dip.

Dinner: Pasta Primavera

What You Will Need:

Spiralized zucchini

Chopped cherry tomatoes, .25 to .5 c

Chopped basil, .25 c

Cayenne, to taste

Sea salt, to taste

Olive oil, .25 c

Thinly sliced red bell pepper

Thinly sliced onion

Sliced yellow squash

Sliced large zucchini

What You Will Do

Add all of the veggies, not including the spiralized zucchini, to a bowl and add in the oil, salt, basil, and pepper. Toss everything together and then spread out on a baking sheet.

Bake the veggies for about 20 minutes, or until they just start to turn brown. If you want, you can sauté your vegetables in some grapeseed oil if you don't want to bake them.

Once the veggies are done, scoop them into a bowl and then add in the spiralized zucchini noodles. Toss everything together so that the zucchini noodles are well coated. Enjoy.

Step-By-Step Guide

A typical day could go like this.

8:00 AM – Start by having a glass of warm lime water. As you are sipping your water, get the ingredients together for your breakfast smoothie.

8:30 AM – Some light exercise for 15 to 30 minutes. Since you are detoxing, you don't want it to be anything extreme or strenuous. A light jog is about as extreme as you want to go. Walking or yoga would be a good idea too.

9:00 AM – Take some time to relax and start writing in your detox journal. It's only been an hour, so you probably haven't experienced any adverse effects from it. You could also write yourself an encouraging note for those rough days. Also, check to see how much water you have drunk so far.

9:30 AM – Fix your breakfast smoothie and take at least a full 30 minutes to sit an enjoy it. You should not watch TV while you are eating.

10:00 AM – If you are taking any supplements, this is the time to take them since you have something on your stomach. Again, check in to make sure you are drinking enough water to reach your goal for a gallon a day.

11:00 AM - Time for your first snack. Now, if at any point during the detox you don't feel like you need a snack, you do not have to eat one and can save it for some other time when do feel like you need. Continue drinking your water for the day.

12:30 PM – It's lunch time. Start making your quinoa and salad. You can enjoy this with a cup of ginger tea if you would like.

1:30 PM – How is your water intake going? If you are feeling tired of water, you can always choose to have an approved herbal tea if you would like to.

2:00 PM – 3:00 PM – Make sure you are drinking plenty of water. If you have some time, you can write in your detox journal again if you are feeling anything different from this morning.

3:30 PM – Time for your second snack. Again, if you don't feel like you need it, then feel free to skip your snack. Continue drinking your water.

4:00 PM – 5:00 PM – Try for a glass of herbal tea to help get your water intake in. The more you drink during the day, the less you will be faced with at the close of the day.

5:30 PM – Time to fix your dinner. Enjoy your pasta primavera and another big glass of water. Your gallon of water for the day should almost be finished.

6:30 PM – 8:30 PM – If you start to feel hungry at any point during the evening, feel free to snack on some of your approved fruits and veggies.

9:00 PM – Bed – Do whatever you want to help you relax for bed. You can have another glass of warm lime water or some herbal tea. Read a book and do some meditation. The important thing is to make sure that you help your body to relax so that it can easily slip off to sleep for the day. Getting a good night's rest will make the next day a lot easier. You can also write in your journal one more time before you go off to sleep.

That's it for day one. Congratulations, you have taken the first step towards reaching the end of your detox. You might be feeling good, or you could be experiencing some side effects. Whichever you may be feeling, sleep well and get ready for day two.

Chapter 6: Detox Day Two

You are getting ready to start day two of your detox. The first day probably seemed like a breeze, you may have already started to struggle a little bit. Today will likely be a bit harder since it will be hitting your body that there has been a lack of food. If you have just given up coffee, you will likely be suffering from a headache. Make sure that you get plenty of water. The water will help to offset some of the side effects since most side effects are due to dehydration. Again, you will find your recipes for the day and well as a guideline for how your day can progress. As always, the guideline is just a suggestion. You can fit what you need to do for the day into the time you have as you see fit as long as you stick to what you are supposed to eat.

Let's not forget to start out day with a glass of warm lime water to help get those toxins moving.

Breakfast: Hemp Seed Porridge

What You Will Need:

Porridge:

Walnut milk, 1 c

Hemp seeds, .5 c

Milk:

Spring water, 4 c

Walnuts, 1 c

What You Will Do:

Let's start by making the walnut milk. Take the walnuts and the spring water and add them to your blender. Mix them together until well blended. It won't be perfectly smooth at this point, but don't worry. Next, you will use a fine mesh sieve or a nut milk bag. Make sure you have a glass jar to catch the milk. Pour the blended walnuts through the strainer to remove any chunks. What you are left with is your walnut milk.

For the porridge, add the hemp seeds and the milk to bowl. Allow this to sit for a little while. You can also add in some herbs and spices from the nutritional guide. A little sprinkling of sea salt helps bring out the natural flavors as well. Some of the best spices to use is ginger and cloves.

Snack 1: Roasted Walnuts

What You Will Need:

Sea salt, 1 tsp

Organic cold pressed olive oil, .25 c

Raw walnuts, 2 c

What You Will Do:

First, you will want to let soak your walnuts before roasting them. Add the walnuts to a bowl and cover them with water. Allow them to soak overnight. Drain the nuts out of the water and lay them on them paper towels to dry a bit.

Next, make sure that you turn your oven to 275. You want to slow roast the walnuts to help them get crunchy.

Add the walnuts into a baggy along with the olive oil and sea salt. Shake the walnuts so that they are all well coated with the oil and salt. Feel free to add any other approved spices here as well. If you want them a bit spicy, cayenne pepper is a good option.

Line a baking sheet with some parchment paper and spread the nuts evenly across the baking sheet. Slide them into the oven and let them bake for 20 minutes.

Once they are done, you can sprinkle them with a bit more salt and then bake for another five minutes. Make sure that before you store them, you allow them to cool off completely. If you seal them into a bowl before they are completely cool, they will start to sweat which will get rid of their crunchiness.

Lunch: Kale Salad with Lime and Avocado Dressing

What You Will Need:

Sea salt

Mashed avocado

Olive oil, .33 c

Lime juice, .5 c

Grated ginger, 2 tsp

Chopped red onion, .5

Dinosaur kale leaves, 5 to 6

What You Will Do:

Let's start by making the dressing. You will add the olive oil, lime juice, and avocado to a bowl. Mash the ingredients together until they form a smooth dressing. Alternatively, you can add the olive oil, lime juice, and avocado to a blender and mix until smooth.

Next, rip the kale leaves up into smaller, more edible, pieces and add them to the bowl containing the dressing. You are going to get your hands a little dirty with this part. Use your hands to massage the dressing into the kale leaves so that the kale isn't so tough.

Next, you can add in all of the other ingredients to the salad and toss everything together. If you want, you can serve the salad over some quinoa and add in some chopped walnuts for some crunch.

Snack 2: Simple Green Juice

What You Will Need:

Lime juice, 4 tbsp

Kale, 5 oz

Wakame, .5 c

Cucumbers, 2

What You Will Do:

If you have a juicer, juice the cucumbers, wakame, and kale together. If you don't have a juicer, you can add the cucumbers, wakame, and kale to a blender and mix until well combined. Then strain the juice through a fine mesh strainer or a nut milk bag. This will make sure that juice is smooth and you won't run into any chunks. Stir in the lime juice and enjoy.

Dinner: Raw Vegan Pad Thai

What You Will Need:

Kelp noodles, 2 bags

Lime juice, to taste

Chopped scallions – garnish

Chopped dill – garnish

Chopped basil – garnish

Minced onion, 1 tsp

Dr. Sebi soy sauce, 2 to 4 tbsp

Minced ginger, 1 tbsp

Fresh orange juice, .5 c

Tahini butter, 1 c

Soy sauce:

Sea moss gel, 1 tsp

Raw agave, 1 tsp

Toasted sesame oil, 2 tsp

Ginger powder, 1 tsp

Sea salt, 1 tbsp

Soaked figs, 5 dried

What You Will Do

Begin by making your soy sauce. You will need to soak the dried figs first. All you need to do is cover them in water and let them soak for at least four hours, or overnight is best. Add the ingredients for the soy sauce to your blender and mix everything together until it forms a sauce. You can taste it and adjust any flavors that you need to.

Next, as you make your pad thai sauce, you will need to soak your kelp noodles. Place the kelp noodles in a bowl and cover them in spring water along with some lime juice. Allow them to soak for at least ten minutes.

Add the minced onion, Dr. Sebi soy sauce, ginger, orange juice, and tahini butter to a blender and mix until smooth. You shouldn't need to add any extra salt.

Drain the water off of the kelp noodles and rinse them under some cool water. Add the noodles into a bowl and then drizzle the sauce over the top. Toss them together and add in a splash of lime juice. Allow this to sit for at least ten minutes so that the kelp noodles soak in all of the flavors.

Sprinkle on the scallions, dill, and basil and enjoy.

Step-By-Step Guide

Since the second and third days tend to be the hardest, sticking to this guide may just help you to stick with your cleanse.

8:00 AM – Start by having a glass of warm lime water. While you are working on your morning cup of tea, get together the ingredients for your breakfast. In fact, you can go ahead and have your hemp seeds soaking.

8:30 AM – Some light exercise for 15 to 30 minutes. Since you are detoxing, you don't want it to be anything extreme or strenuous. A light jog is about as extreme as you want to go, especially if you are feeling any side effects. Walking or yoga would be a good idea too. There are a lot of yoga routines that can aid in detoxing. If you don't feel like doing a workout, which is okay since a lot is going on for your body right now, you can do a little meditation to help you get yourself into the right head space. Having some things to do that will distract you from the detox and help to offset any side effects that you may be experiencing.

9:00 AM – Take some time to relax and start writing in your detox journal. Since you are an hour into your second day, you have probably experienced some things, good and bad. Make sure you keep up with these experiences in your journal so that you can look back and see how far you have come. You also need to check to see how you are doing on your water intake.

9:30 AM – Now you can enjoy your hemp seed porridge. You can have a glass of herbal tea with breakfast if you would like. As always, make sure your food has your full attention. When you focus fully on your food, it will help you to feel fuller because every part of your body will know you are eating.

Eating slowly also helps. Eating too fast is one of the main causes of weight gain because people don't allow their stomachs enough time to let their brain know they are full, so they go back for seconds even though they probably didn't need to.

10:00 AM – If you are taking any supplements, this is the time to take them since you have something on your stomach. Depending on if you are on any prescriptions, when you take your supplements may change. The main thing is to make sure you don't take supplements on an empty stomach, and that you take them an hour before prescriptions. Again, check in to make sure you are drinking enough water to reach your goal for a gallon a day.

11:00 AM - Time for your first snack. Remember, if you don't feel like you need a snack at this point, then don't worry about eating a snack. It will always be there for you should you feel like you need one. Continue drinking your water for the day.

11:15 AM – 12:15 AM – This time be used to do whatever you want. If you are working while doing your detox, then you will likely have that to keep you occupied, which will make your detox go by a bit easier.

12:30 PM – It's lunch time. Get working on that tasty kale salad and enjoy every bite of it. You can enjoy this with a cup of ginger tea if you would like or you can have a glass of bromide plus.

1:30 PM – How is your water intake going? If you are feeling tired of water, you can always choose to have an approved herbal tea if you would like to. Since it's midday, I would avoid going with chamomile.

2:00 PM – 3:00 PM – Make sure you are drinking plenty of water. If you have some time, you can write in your detox journal again if you are feeling anything different from this morning.

3:30 PM – Time for your second snack. Again, if you don't feel like you need it, then feel free to skip your snack. Continue drinking your water.

4:00 PM – 5:00 PM – Try for a glass of herbal tea to help get your water intake in. The more water you get out of the way during the day, the less you will have to worry with during your evening.

5:30 PM – Time to fix your dinner. Enjoy having that pad thai knowing that it is nourishing your body. Make sure you rinse it down with a glass of water. Your gallon of water for the day should almost be finished.

6:30 PM – 8:30 PM – If you start to feel hungry at any point during the evening feel free to snack on some of your approved fruits and veggies. Also, now is the time to enjoy a glass of chamomile tea to help you start winding down for bed.

9:00 PM – Bed – Do whatever you want to help you relax for bed. You can have another glass of warm lime water or some herbal tea. Read a book and do some meditation. The important thing is to make sure that you help your body to relax so that it can easily slip off to sleep for the day. Getting a good night's rest will make the next day a lot easier. You can also write in your journal one more time before you go off to sleep.

You've officially finished day two. You should be feeling pretty good about yourself. Today may have been a bit harder than yesterday, and that's okay. This is normal for a detox because your body is not getting the addictive substances that it is used to. Right now your body may be freaking out, but reassure yourself that you are doing the right thing. You are nourishing your body, and the in the coming days, those bad feelings you have been having will go away. One day, you will wake up feeling better than you have ever felt before. Pushing through the side effects is one of the best things you can do for your body.

Chapter 7: Detox Day Three

You've reached day three of your detox. Day three, for most, tends to be the day when the majority of changes will happen to your body. This makes the day particularly harder, and a lot of people have reported that the third day is when most of the mucus is cleared out. Depending on how you ate before you began your cleanse, and how well you prepped, today or tomorrow could be your hardest day. Either way, don't be surprised if you feel bad on day three. If it is at all possible, it would be a good idea to take the day off so that you can relax and let your body do what it needs to. As always, all of your recipes are below along with a guideline to follow for your day.

Let's not forget to start out day with a glass of warm lime water to help get those toxins moving.

Breakfast: Quinoa with Walnut Milk

What You Will Need:

Coconut oil, 1 tbsp

Spring water, .5 c

Walnut milk, 1.5 c

Cloves, .25 tsp

Ginger, .25 tsp

Quinoa, .5 c

What You Will Do:

This will use some of the milk that you made the day before. If you don't have any leftover, make sure that you make a fresh batch. Store-bought nut milks are not a good option because they have a lot of different additives.

To start your breakfast, add a pot over medium and add in the quinoa, cloves, and ginger. Stir the quinoa around and toast it for about two to three minutes. This will help bring out all of its natural flavors and give it a nice nutty taste. You will want to stir it frequently so that it does not end up burning.

Next, add in the spring water and walnut milk. Allow the mixture to come up to a boil and then allow it to simmer for about 25 minutes. The quinoa should be tender and it should be about the consistency of porridge. If it isn't soft, add a bit more water and let it continue to cook for a bit longer. Make sure that you stir it occasionally so that it does not end up burning.

Once it is cooked, stir in the coconut oil until melted and add a sprinkling of sea salt to bring out its natural flavors.

Snack 1: Banana Chips

What You Will Need:

Favorite Dr. Sebi approved seasonings

Green burro bananas, 3

Olive oil, 2 tbsp

What You Will Do:

For these to work right, you will have to make sure that you have green burro bananas. The bananas are firmer and will hold their shape and get crunchier than if the banana is ripe. It also isn't as sweet, so it works well if you want a savory treat, but it does well with sweet flavorings as well.

You will need to start by making sure that you oven is at 450. Add some parchment paper to a baking sheet and set to the side as you prepare the bananas.

Peel the bananas, making sure that you remove all of the strings. Slice the bananas up into quarter-inch thick slices. Since it is a green banana it should be easier to slice and they shouldn't mush-up in your hand. Make sure that you pull the banana pieces apart and lay them flat across the prepared baking sheet.

For a savory chip: Mix together the olive oil with some sea salt, cayenne pepper, basil, oregano, and onion powder until well combined. Brush the tops of the bananas with the oil mixture. Bake the bananas for eight minutes. Remove them from the oven and then flip the bananas over. Brush the other side with the rest of the oil mixture and then bake for another seven minutes.

For a sweet chip: Mix together the olive oil with some date sugar, sea salt, cloves, ginger, and sweet basil until well combined. Brush the tops of the bananas with the sugar mixture and bake them for about eight minutes. Tape them out of the oven and flip the bananas over, brushing the other side with the rest of the mixture. Bake for another seven minutes, or until they have reached your desired crunchiness.

You will want to make sure that the bananas are completely cool before you store them in a container. If they are still warm when stored, they will start to sweat which will cause them to lose their crunchiness

Lunch: Romaine Lettuce Wraps

What You Will Need:

Chickpeas – optional

Chopped fresh basil

Plum tomato

Chopped cucumber, .5

An avocado

Romaine lettuce leaves, 3 to 4

Walnut Hummus Variation:

Tahini, .24 c

Spring water, 1 tbsp

Cayenne pepper, .25 tsp

Onion powder, 1.5 tsp

Sea salt, 1.25 tsp

Sage, 1 tsp

Raw walnuts that have be soaked for at least eight hours and dried, 1.25 c

Lime juice, .25 c

Olive oil, 3 tbsp

Grated ginger, 2 tbsp

Chopped zucchini, 2 c

What You Will Do:

If you want to have chickpeas with your meal, you will want to make sure that you soak them and cook them before you enjoy them.

For the avocado version: Take your avocado and mash it up. You can mix in some salt and lime juice if you would like to give it a little more flavor. Chop up your tomato and half of a cucumber as well. Spread the each of the romaine leaves with some of the mashed avocado. Top the avocado with some cucumber, chickpeas, tomato, and fresh basil. You can also add in any other approved veggies if you would like. Add a little lime juice and salt for extra flavor.

For the walnut hummus version: Start by adding the lime juice, olive oil, ginger, and zucchini to a blender. Mix until smooth. Add in the walnuts and blend everything together until it becomes smooth again. Add in the remaining ingredients, minus the tahini, and mix until combined. Lastly, mix in the tahini. To build the lettuce wraps, spread the walnut hummus across the lettuce and top with the vegetables and chickpeas from above.

Snack 2: Vegetables with Walnut Hummus

What You Will Need:

Leftover walnut hummus from lunch

Sliced cucumbers

Sliced bell pepper

Sliced zucchini

What You Will Do:

For today's midday snack, you will need some of the walnut hummus that you used for your lunch wraps. Then pick some of your favorite approved veggies, cucumbers, zucchini, and bell peppers work best, and dip them into the hummus and enjoy.

Dinner: "Tuna" Salad

What You Will Need:

Lime juice, 1tbso

Dulse flakes, 1.5 tbsp

Chopped fresh savory, 2 tbsp

Chopped fresh dill, 2 tbsp

Finely chopped onion, 2 tbsp

Finely chopped olives, .25 c

Sea salt, .5 tsp

Olive oil, 1.5 tbsp

Raw chickpeas, 1.5 c

What You Will Do

The first thing you need to do is to get your chickpeas ready. Add the chickpeas to a bowl and cover them with cold water. Place them in the refrigerator and allow them to soak overnight. When you drain the water off the next morning, you can save the water. This is known as aquafaba and can be used in various different ways. You can also use it in recipes that call for regular spring water to add an extra layer of flavor.

Drain the water off of the chickpeas and the rinse them in some cool water. Add the chickpeas to a pot and cover them with water again. Allow the water to come up to a boil and then turn it down so that they are simmering. Watch the boiling process because chickpeas will form a foam. Skim it off of the top when it forms and turn the heat down a bit. Chickpeas will typically take about an hour to an hour and a half to cook. It's a good idea to have some cooked chickpeas made up before your detox begins.

Add the cooked and cooled chickpeas to a bowl and mash them up with a fork. Add all of the other ingredients to the chickpeas and continue to stir and mash the mixture together. Do this until it starts to look like tuna.

This can be served as a wrap in some romaine lettuce leaves, or you can serve it over top of a salad. You can also eat it on its own or with some spelt crackers.

Step-By-Step Guide

Since the second and third days tend to be the hardest, sticking to this guide may just help you to stick with your cleanse.

8:00 AM – Start by having a glass of warm lime water. While you are working on your morning cup of tea, gather everything you need for your quinoa porridge this morning. I won't start cooking it just yet.

8:30 AM – Some light exercise for 15 to 30 minutes. Today is likely another tough day since your body will be getting rid of a lot of toxins today, so it is okay if you don't feel good enough to do an actual workout. If all you can muster is a short walk, then that is perfectly okay for your body at this point. If you want, you can also simply to a quick meditation to help center your mind. The goal is to work your body or mind in some way so that you detox every part of your body and not just your gut.

9:00 AM – Take some time to relax and start writing in your detox journal. Since you are an hour into your third day, you have probably experienced some things, good and bad. This may be the worst day of your detox, so you really need to lean into your journaling and mental health work.

9:30 AM – Now you can enjoy your quinoa porridge. You can have a glass of herbal tea with breakfast if you would like. As always, make sure your food has your full attention. Think about how the food is nourishing your body in ways that we can't fully understand. Notice how the porridge tastes and feels. Doing this will help you appreciate your food for what it does for you, instead of simply being something you do to fill your time.

10:00 AM – If you are taking any supplements, this is the time to take them since you have something on your stomach. When you take your supplements, you should try to take them with an entire glass of water to make sure you get them washed down.

Again, check in to make sure you are drinking enough water to reach your goal for a gallon a day.

11:00 AM - Time for your first snack. Really get into the act of cooking your food. This takes your mind of any struggles you may be having. Today, more than any other day, you will likely be looking forward to this snack. Make sure you drink a glass of water with your snack as well.

11:15 AM – 12:15 PM – This time be used to do whatever you want. If you are working while doing your detox, then you will likely have that to keep you occupied, which will make your detox go by a bit easier. If you don't have anything to do, you may feel like taking a bit of a nap right now.

12:30 PM – It's lunch time. Get working on that tasty romaine lettuce wrap. Remember, you have two choices for today's lunch. Enjoy every bite of whichever version you decided to enjoy. You can enjoy this with a cup of fennel tea if you would like or you can have a glass of bromide plus.

1:30 PM – How is your water intake going? If you are feeling tired of water, you can always choose to have an approved herbal tea if you would like to. Pick a tea that can give that pick-me-up that you may need right now.

2:00 PM – 3:00 PM – Make sure you are drinking plenty of water. If you have some time, you can write in your detox journal again if you are feeling anything different from this morning.

3:30 PM – Time for your second snack. Again, if you don't feel like you need it, then feel free to skip your snack. Continue drinking your water.

4:00 PM – 5:00 PM – Try for a glass of herbal tea to help get your water intake in. The more water you get out of the way during the day, the less you will have to worry with during your evening.

5:30 PM – Time to fix your dinner. Enjoy having that "tuna" salad knowing that it is providing your body with lots of healthy nutrients. Make sure you rinse it down with a glass of water. Your gallon of water for the day should almost be finished.

6:30 PM – 8:30 PM – If you start to feel hungry at any point during the evening feel free to snack on some of your approved fruits and veggies. Also, now is the time to enjoy a glass of chamomile tea to help you start winding down for bed.

9:00 PM – Bed – Do whatever you want to help you relax for bed. You can have another glass of warm lime water or some herbal tea. Read a book and do some meditation. The important thing is to make sure that you help your body to relax so that it can easily slip off to sleep for the day. Getting a good night's rest will make the next day a lot easier. You can also write in your journal one more time before you go off to sleep.

You've made it through day three. If at any point during the day you felt like giving up, that's okay because you pushed through anyway. Today was probably hard, so you should be very proud of yourself for what you have accomplished. The following days should get a bit easier. That said, some people may find that day four is just as hard or harder than day three, but trust me, it won't be this hard for much longer. Your body is flushing out the remaining bits of toxins it has held onto for years. Soon, your body will be rebuilding your cells and you will start to have more energy than ever before.

Chapter 8: Detox Day Four

You are getting ready to start day four of your detox. As mentioned in day three, today could be another rough day for you depending on how you prepared. Heavy coffee drinkers and sugar users will likely find that today is just as bad as yesterday, and that is totally okay. Everybody is different so everybody's experience is going to be different. The important thing is to remember you are doing a great service to your body, and you will get through this. As always, the recipes you need for the day are below along with a step-by-step guideline for the day.

Let's not forget to start our day with a glass of warm lime water to help get those toxins moving.

Breakfast: Avocado on Toast

What You Will Need:

Cayenne pepper, to taste

Slice of spelt bread, or any bread made by Dr. Sebi approved grains

Juice of half a lime

Extra virgin olive oil, 1 tsp

A ripe avocado

What You Will Do:

This is a quick and easy breakfast. The first thing you need to do is mash the avocado up in a bowl along with the cayenne, olive oil, and lime juice. Spread the mashed avocado over the toast and enjoy. Feel free to toast your bread first if you would like. You can also simple slice the avocado up and place it on the bread and sprinkle it with the rest of the ingredients.

Snack 1: Roasted Walnuts

What You Will Need:

Sea salt

Grapeseed oil

Bundle of dinosaur kale

What You Will Do:

Start by ripping the kale leaves off of their stem. Rip them into smaller chip-sized pieces and then place them into a bowl. Add in some oil and salt and toss them altogether.

Spread the kale over a baking sheet. Make sure that you have your oven at 350. Bake your kale chips for 15 minutes. Enjoy

Lunch: Wild Rice with Nopales and Tamarind

What You Will Need:

Sea salt

Cayenne pepper

Sesame seeds, .5 c

Grated ginger, 1 tsp

Agave nectar, 2 tsp

Tamarind, 2 tsp

Zest of a lime

Lime juice, .5 c

Thinly sliced scallions, 4

Nopales paddle

Wild rice, 1 c

Spring water, 2 c

What You Will Do:

Start by bring the two cups of water to a boil. You can salt the water a bit, if you would like, to help season the wild rice. Once boiling, add in the rice, turn the heat down, place on the lid, and let the rice cook for 25 to 30 minutes or until soft and the water has been absorbed.

Next you will need to get your nopales ready. When you are picking out your nopales paddles, you want ones that are flexible but aren't completely soft. They need to give a little but not a lot. The smaller paddles tend to be more tender.

You will need to cut the knobs and spines off. Using a peeler or a knife make gentle and shallow sawing motions across the nopales. Try to leave as much of the skin on it as you can and just cut off the spines and knobs. This works best if you hold your knife perpendicular to the nopales and scrape inwards. Next, cut about a quarter of an inch off of the edges and the slice a half of an inch off of the base. Wash the nopales and the slice it into strips.

Next, add some grapeseed oil to a skillet and heat. Add in the nopales along with a bit of sea salt and cook them for a few minutes. Turn the heat down and place a lid on the pan. Allow the nopales to sweat for about 20 minutes, or until you notice that the clear substances has cooked away.

As the nopales is cooking, beat together the ginger, agave, tamarind, lime zest, and lime juice. When the nopales are just about finished, add in the scallions and cook until soft.

Once the rice is cooked, add in the napoles and scallions and mix together. Pour in the lime juice mixture and toss everything together. Season with some sea salt and cayenne for flavor and top it with the sesame seeds.

Snack 2: Simple Green Juice

What You Will Need:

Lime juice, 4 tbsp

Dandelion green, 5 oz

Nori, .5 c

Cucumbers, 2

What You Will Do:

If you have a juicer, juice the cucumbers, nori, and dandelion greens together. If you don't have a juicer, you can add the cucumbers, nori, and dandelion greens to a blender and mix until well combined. Then strain the juice through a fine mesh strainer or a nut milk bag. This will make sure that juice is smooth and you won't run into any chunks. Stir in the lime juice and enjoy.

Dinner: Raw Vegan Pad Thai

What You Will Need:

Sea salt

Chopped sage leaves, 1 handful

Homemade vegetable stock, 2.5 c

Wild rice, 1 c

Grated ginger, 2 tsp

Chopped red onion

Extra virgin olive oil, 3 tbsp

Sliced butternut squash, 7 oz

What You Will Do

You will start by getting your oven to 350. As your oven is heating up, work on slicing up your butternut squash and then place it evenly across a parchment lined baking sheet. Drizzle the squash with two tablespoons of your extra virgin olive oil. Place this in the oven and let it bake for 15 minutes. The squash should be very soft to the point that it becomes creamy when pressed.

In a pan, add the rest of the extra virgin olive oil. Add the onion and the grated ginger to your pan. Allow these to cook, while stirring constantly, for a minute. Add in the wild rice, still constantly stirring, for another minute to toast the rice a bit.

Add in two ladles of your homemade vegetable stock to your wild rice. Allow the rice to simmer for awhile until it has absorbed all of the stock. Make sure that you stir it frequently. Once the stock has been absorbed, add another ladle full of stock to the rice. Continue to do this until the wild rice has become soft and is cooked through. Once the rice has been cooking for about 30 minutes, add the chopped sage leaves and the cooked butternut squash.

You will continue the additions of vegetable stock to the rice mixture until the rice has become soft and cooked through. Make sure that you stir it often. This will take about 50 minutes in total. Once the rice is cooked, serve and enjoy.

Step-By-Step Guide

You've probably gotten the hand of how your day is going to go by this point, but as always, here is a guideline for your day four.

8:00 AM – Start by having a glass of warm lime water. As you are enjoying your tea, you can gather together you breakfast ingredients. You could go ahead and make your avocado toast, just make sure that you use plenty of lime juice so that the avocado doesn't turn brown.

8:30 AM – Some light exercise for 15 to 30 minutes. Since you're right in the middle of your detox, this could be your worst day or you could be feeling better by this point. Depending on how you are feeling, you could opt for a simple meditation to work your and cleanse your mind, you could be feeling up to a light jog around the block or a vigorous yoga workout. Listen to your body to see what it wants you to do.

9:00 AM – Take some time to relax and start writing in your detox journal. You're at your fourth day so you have probably had a quite a few different experiences. You can even look back over your past journal entries to see how things have changed.

9:30 AM – Now you can enjoy your avocado toast. You can have a glass of herbal tea with breakfast if you would like. Make sure that you are paying attention to your food as you eat. While I don't remind you to do this with every meal you eat, you should be. Watching TV as you eat causes mindless eating. You want mindful eating. Be aware of your food, how it tastes, and what it is doing for your body.

10:00 AM – If you are taking any supplements, this is the time to take them since you have something on your stomach. Make sure that you wash your supplements down with plenty of water. Again, check in to make sure you are drinking enough water to reach your goal for a gallon a day.

11:00 AM - Time for your first snack. Remember, if you don't feel like you need a snack at this point, then don't worry about eating a snack. It will always be there for you should you feel like you need one. Continue drinking your water for the day.

11:15 AM – 12:15 AM – This time be used to do whatever you want. If you are working while doing your detox, then you will likely have that to keep you occupied, which will make your detox go by a bit easier. You may also feel like taking some time for yourself right now depending on how your experience is going.

12:30 PM – It's lunch time. Now is the time to enjoy your wild rice with nopales. If you have never had cactus before, you are in for a real treat. You could also try having a glass of tamarind tea to go with this, or simple a glass of water.

1:30 PM – How is your water intake going? If you are feeling tired of water, you can always choose to have an approved herbal tea if you would like to. Try some raspberry tea to help you through the afternoon.

2:00 PM – 3:00 PM – Make sure you are drinking plenty of water. If you have some time, you can write in your detox journal again if you are feeling anything different from this morning. If things are rough for you, look back over your journal and find some encouragement.

3:30 PM – Time for your second snack. Again, if you don't feel like you need it, then feel free to skip your snack. Continue drinking your water.

4:00 PM – 5:00 PM – Try for a glass of herbal tea to help get your water intake in. The more water you get out of the way during the day, the less you will have to worry with during your evening.

5:30 PM – Time to fix your dinner. Enjoy having that butternut squash risotto. Make sure you rinse it down with a glass of water. Your gallon of water for the day should almost be finished.

6:30 PM – 8:30 PM – If you start to feel hungry at any point during the evening feel free to snack on some of your approved fruits and veggies. Also, now is the time to enjoy a glass of chamomile tea to help you start winding down for bed.

9:00 PM – Bed – Do whatever you want to help you relax for bed. You can have another glass of warm lime water or some herbal tea. Read a book and do some meditation. The important thing is to make sure that you help your body to relax so that it can easily slip off to sleep for the day. Getting a good night's rest will make the next day a lot easier. You can also write in your journal one more time before you go off to sleep.

You've made it to the end of day four. You are over halfway done with your cleanse. That's a big step, and the rest of the days should be downhill from now. Your body has done a lot of adapting, and most of the toxins should all be cleaned from your cells by now. You have likely noticed a loss of mucus. You may have even noticed other changes in your body, like a reduction in aches and pains, or you may have noticed a little more energy. The last few days of the detox should go a lot easier than the first few.

Chapter 9: Detox Day Five

You've made it to the fifth day of your detox. You should be feeling pretty good about yourself right now. Your side effects should be nonexistent by now and you might have noticed some pounds have been lost. You might also notice your gut health and overall body health is doing better, too. You might notice you're your energy levels are up. You should be proud of yourself you are almost to the end if your journey. You will find the recipes for today below. Just continue to do what you've been doing and you will feel like you have a brand new body.

Remember to start your day with a glass of warm lime water. To help get rid of all those toxins.

Breakfast: Kamut Cereal

What You Will Need:

Soft jelly coconut, 1 tbsp

Raisins, .5 c

Cloves, 1 tsp

Sesame seeds, .25 c

Hemp seeds, .25 c

Walnuts, .5 c

Puffed kamut, .75 c

What You Will Do:

Start by soaking the walnuts in some water overnight. The next morning, drain well. Place the soft jelly coconut, raisins, cloves, sesame seeds, hemp seeds, walnuts, and puffed kamut into a bowl and mix well.

You can serve this either hot or cold with some coconut milk.

Snack 1: Kale Chips

What You Will Need:

Sea salt

Grapeseed oil

Bundle of dinosaur kale

What You Will Do:

You need to warm your oven to 350.

Begin by washing the kale and ripping the leaves off the stems. Tear them into smaller bite size pieces and put them into a bowl. Add some oil and salt and toss them together.

Line a baking sheet with a piece of parchment paper. Place the kale evenly over the baking sheet. Place inside the oven and bake for 15 minutes.

Carefully remove from oven and enjoy.

Lunch: Quinoa Vegetable Soup

What You Will Need:

Chopped basil, 4 tbsp

Dr. Sebi soy sauce, 2 tsp (refer to day 2 dinner recipes)

Juice of two key limes

Chopped onions, 1 medium

Soursop leaves, 2 c

Spring water, 1 c

Homemade vegetable stock, 1 c

Quinoa, 1 c

What You Will Do:

Pour the vegetable stock into a pot. Add the quinoa and bring it to a boil. Once boiling, turn heat down to a simmer. Continue to cook for 20 minutes. You don't need to put a lid on the pot. If all the liquid gets absorbed before the quinoa is cooked, add some more water. Once quinoa is cooked through, fluff with fork and set to the side.

In another pot, add one cup water and bring the water to a full rolling boil. Add in the onion, soursop leaves, lime juice, and Dr. Sebi soy sauce. Turn the heat down and simmer for about five minutes.

Add the amount of quinoa you want in your soup into the pot with the vegetables. When ready, ladle into a soup bowl and garnish with basil. Enjoy.

Snack 2: Veggies and Guacamole

What You Will Need:

Sea salt, to taste

Juice of one key lime

Ground oregano, .5 tsp

Chopped tomato, .5 small

Chopped red onion, .25 c

Avocado, 1 large

Sliced bell pepper

Sliced cucumber

What You Will Do:

Slice the avocado lengthwise and twist to separate. Carefully remove the pit and scoop the flesh out into a bowl. Using a fork, mash the avocado until chunky. Add in the lime juice, onion, tomato, and seasonings. Stir well to combine.

Enjoy with sliced vegetables.

Dinner: Layered Vegetable Bake

What You Will Need:

Zucchini, 2 medium

Butternut squash

Water, 2 tbsp

Oregano, pinch

Onion powder, 1 tsp

Dr. Sebi soy sauce, .5 tsp

Sliced onion, 1

Chopped Roma tomatoes, 5

Avocado oil, 4 tbsp

Quinoa, .5 c

What You Will Do

You need to warm your oven to 340.

Put the quinoa into a small pot and cover with some water. Bring to a full rolling boil. Turn down heat to a simmer and cook for 15 minutes. Set this to the side.

Put the avocado oil into a large skillet. Put the tomatoes into the oil and mash and make a base for your sauce. You can do with a potato masher or fork.

Add onion, oregano, onion powder, and "soy sauce". Add water and continue to cook until it has reduced to a thick sauce.

While this is cooking, prep your zucchini and butternut squash. You need to slice the zucchini lengthwise into thin strips. Cut the butternut squash in half and scoop out the seeds. Slice this as thin as possible lengthwise.

Add the quinoa and just a bit more water. Simmer for five more minutes.

You now need to layer your vegetables. Place half of the butternut squash into the bottom of a baking dish. Add about one third of the zucchini on top.

Spread about half of the quinoa mixture on top.

Continue with these layers until you finish with zucchini on top.

Brush the top of the zucchini with some avocado oil and put into your preheated oven for 45 minutes until vegetables are tender.

Step-By-Step Guide

A typical day could go like this.

8:00 AM – This is your fifth day so you probably know how your day is going to go. You will begin by having your glass of warm lime water. As you are sipping your water, get the ingredients together for your breakfast cereal. If you want, you can go ahead and mix everything together so the kamut can soak in the milk.

8:30 AM – Get 15 to 30 minutes of exercise in. Since you are likely feeling better than you have over the last couple of days, you can start doing more in your workout. You may even feel like going for a light jog or upping your yoga routine to something that is a little more strenuous than what you have been doing. Feel free to meditate during this time as well if you would like. Remember, a mental cleanse is just as important as physical one.

9:00 AM – Take some time to relax and write some things out in your detox journal. Now would be a good time to look back over your journey and see how you have been doing. You likely aren't feeling a lot in the way of side effects, and if you are, they shouldn't be as bad as they were the last two days. You are probably feelings pretty good about yourself. Put all of these feelings and emotions into your journal. Check on the amount of water you have drunk today and grab a glass if you need to. Remember if you feel a headache coming on, you might not be getting enough water.

9:30 AM – Fix your breakfast cereal and take at least a full 30 minutes to sit an enjoy it. Remember to always pay attention to your food. When you are fully focused on your food, it can help you feel fuller since every part of your body knows that you are eating. Remember to eat slowly because it can help with this too. When we eat fast, it can cause us to gain weight because we aren't letting our stomachs have enough time to tell our brains that we are full. You might even think you need more to eat when you really don't.

10:00 AM – If you are taking any supplements, this is the time to take them since you have something on your stomach. It wouldn't hurt to have a cup of bromide tea as well. Again, check in to make sure you are drinking enough water to reach your goal for a gallon a day.

11:00 AM - Time for your first snack. Since you have worked over the hump, you may not need a snack at this time. You can do whatever you feel like you need to. Remember to listen to your body. If you feel like you need this snack, by all means eat it. You might not want it now but might feel a bit hungry later on. That is fine. Just eat when your body tells you it needs it. Continue drinking your water for the day.

11: 15 AM – 12:15 PM – During this time you can do whatever you want. Give yourself a treat, not food though, because you have been rocking this detox. Find something fun to do. Call up a friend and go to the mall. Sit and have a good laugh. Take some water with you to make sure you are getting all you need.

12:30 PM – It's lunch time. Start making your quinoa vegetable soup. You can enjoy your meal with a cup of fennel tea if you would like to. At any point during the day, you can have another cup of warm lime water as well.

1:30 PM – How is your water intake going? If you are feeling tired of water, you can always choose to have an approved herbal tea if you would like to.

2:00 PM – 3:00 PM – Again check your water level and make sure you are drinking plenty of water. If you have some time, you can write in your detox journal about the progress you have made on this journey.

3:30 PM – Time for your second snack. Again, if you don't feel like you need it, then feel free to skip your snack. Continue drinking your water.

4:00 PM – 5:00 PM – Try for a glass of herbal tea to help get your water intake in. The more you drink during the day, the less you will be faced with at the close of the day.

5:30 PM – Time to fix your dinner. Enjoy your layered vegetable bake and another big glass of water. Your gallon of water for the day should almost be finished.

6:30 PM – 8:30 PM – If you start to feel hungry at any point during the evening, feel free to snack on some of your approved fruits and veggies.

9:00 PM – Bed – Do whatever you want to help you relax for bed. You can have another glass of warm lime water or some herbal tea. Read a book and do some meditation. The important thing is to make sure that you help your body to relax so that it can easily slip off to sleep for the day. Getting a good night's rest will make the next day a lot easier. You can also write in your journal one more time before you go off to sleep.

That's it. You've finished another day on your detox journey. Keep it up you only have two more days to go. Things have likely gotten a lot easier, and you are probably glad you pushed through those hard times during the last couple of days. There may still be times when it feels tough, but notice how your body is feeling. There are probably a lot of differences in your body that you have started to notice. Your skin may seem clearer and brighter and you may have a pep in your step that you have never had before. Remind yourself of those wins whenever things feel tough. It won't be much longer now, and you will be completely finished with your detox and brand new version of yourself.

Chapter 10: Detox Day Six

You are on day six of you detox and you are probably feeling pretty good about yourself. Your body is probably thanking you right now. You might not have been feeling any side effects for a few days now. You might be feeling more energetic and want to do more things and this is great news. You will find the recipes for today below. Just continue to do what you've been doing and you will feel like you have a brand new body.

Remember to start your day with a glass of warm lime water. To help get rid of all those toxins.

Breakfast: Breakfast Burrito

What You Will Need:

Olive oil, 1 tsp

Sea salt, .75 tsp

Ginger, 1.5 tsp

Cayenne, pinch

Onion powder, 1 tsp

Cooked and smashed chickpeas, 1 c

Chopped onion, .5 c

Diced mushrooms, 1 c

Diced bell pepper, .75 c

Grapeseed oil, 2 tbsp

For the wrap:

Amaranth greens, 1 c

2 to 4 Dr. Sebi approved wraps

What You Will Do:

You need to start by cooking the chickpeas. Once they are soft enough, you need to smash them. Now prep the rest of your vegetables. Take the peel off the onion and dice it up. Cut the top off the bell pepper and remove the ribs and seeds and dice it up. Wipe the mushrooms with a damp paper towel and dice them up.

Warm the olive oil in a skillet and add the bell pepper, mushrooms, and onions and cook until vegetables begin to soften. Add in the chickpeas and continue to cook until chickpeas are heated through.

Add in amaranth greens just long enough to wilt it. Take off heat.

You can warm your wraps in another dry skillet over low heat. When ready to assemble, divide your chickpea mixture evenly between the wraps. You can serve warm with some homemade guacamole or salsa on the side.

Snack 1: Roasted Walnuts

What You Will Need:

Sea salt, 1 tsp

Avocado oil, .25 c

Raw walnuts, 2 c

What You Will Do:

You need to warm your oven to 275.

Put the walnuts in a baggy. Pour in the avocado oil and shake to coat.

Spread the walnuts over a baking sheet. When the oven has preheated, place the baking sheet into the oven and cook for 20 minutes.

Carefully take the walnuts out of the oven and sprinkle with salt. Put them back into the oven for five minutes.

You can enjoy these warm if you would like. You need to let them cool completely before you put them into a glass jar.

If you put the warm walnuts into a glass jar, it will cause them to sweat and they won't be crunchy anymore. You can get creative with your spices. If you want your walnuts to be a bit more spicy, sprinkle on some cayenne pepper and give them a squirt of lime juice.

Lunch: Fennel and Portobello Mushroom Salad

What You Will Need:

Chopped tarragon, handful

Sesame seeds, .5 tbsp

Juice of one key lime

Fennel bulb

Avocado oil, 2 tbsp

Sea salt, pinch

Thyme, 3 sprigs

Diced onion, 1 small

Portobello mushroom, 1

What You Will Do:

You need to begin by warming your oven to 350.

Wipe the mushrooms off with a damp paper towel. Place it on a baking sheet. Sprinkle with salt, thyme, and onion. Drizzle with one tablespoon of the avocado oil.

Place into the oven and cook for 15 minutes.

While the mushroom is baking, wash the fennel, remove the tops and dice the bulb into bite size pieces. Place into a bowl and drizzle with lime juice and the rest of the avocado oil. Wash the tarragon and chop finely for serving.

When ready to serve: Put the mushroom on a plate. Top with the fennel mixture. Sprinkle on some sesame seeds and the chopped tarragon.

Snack 2: Green Juice

What You Will Need:

Ginger root, 1 tbsp

Tarragon, .5 c

Key lime juice, 4 tbsp

Kale, large handful

Dandelion greens, 1 c

Cucumbers, 2

What You Will Do:

Wash the kale and dandelion greens and give them a rough chop. Roughly chop the cucumber. Peel the ginger root and slice it into small slices.

Put all of this into your blender except lime juice. Turn the blender on and let it run until you have a creamy and smooth juice.

Pour this through a cheese cloth or fine strainer to catch all the pulp. Give the cheesecloth a good squeeze to get all the juice out.

Pour into a glass bottle or Mason jar. Add in the lime juice and give it a good stir. Enjoy.

Dinner: Veggie Pizza

What You Will Need:

For Crust:

Spring water, 1 c

Grapeseed oil, 2 tsp

Agave, 2 tsp

Sea salt, 1 tsp

Oregano, 1 tsp

Onion powder, 1 tsp

Spelt flour, 1.5 c

For Tomato Sauce:

Basil, pinch

Grapeseed oil, 2 tbsp

Agave, 2 tbsp

Oregano, 1 tsp

Onion powder, 1 tsp

Sea salt, 1 tsp

Chopped onion, 2 tbsp

Roma tomatoes, 5

Toppings:

Sliced onions

Sliced bell peppers

Sliced mushrooms

Brazil nut cheese

What You Will Do

For Crust:

You need to begin by warming your oven to 400.

Place the ingredients for the crust into a mixing bowl only adding in half of a cup of water. Add the water in very slowly until the dough can be formed into a ball. You can add more water if you used too much flour.

Take your baking sheet and lightly coat it with some grapeseed oil. Coat your hands with some flour. And press the dough out onto the baking sheet.

Brush the crust with more grapeseed oil and using a fork to poke some holes into the dough. Place the dough into the oven and bake for about 15 minutes.

While the crust is baking, you can prepare the tomato sauce and your vegetables.

Put a pot of water on the stove to boil.

To make it easier to peel the tomato, cut a small "X" on the end of the tomatoes and put them in the boiling water for just one minute.

After one minute, carefully remove the tomatoes with a slotted spoon and put them into a bowl of ice water for about 30 seconds. You will be able to easily peel the skin off.

Place them into your blender along with the basil, grapeseed oil, agave, oregano, onion powder, salt, and chopped onion. Turn the blender on and let it run for about 30 seconds until it is smooth.

Peel and thinly slice the onion. Cut the top off the bell pepper and remove ribs and seeds, thinly slice. Wipe the mushrooms with a damp paper towel and thinly slice. Set all these to the side until ready to use.

Once your pizza crust is done, carefully remove it from the oven and smear with the tomato sauce. Sprinkle on some Brazil nut cheese** and layer on the vegetables any way you would like.

Place the pizza back into the oven and bake an additional 20 minutes.

You will notice that I didn't give you any quantities for the vegetables. This is because only you know how many vegetables you like on your pizza. You can even substitute the vegetables for any of Dr. Sebi's approved veggies like kale, olives, zucchini, avocado, etc.

**The nut cheese will help the topping to cook while baking. If you don't have nut cheese, you will need to sauté the vegetables a bit before you putting them on the pizza. This will keep them from being so raw.

Step-By-Step Guide

A typical day could go like this.

8:00 AM – This is almost your last day so you probably know how your day is going to go. You will begin by having your glass of warm lime water. As you are sipping your water, get the ingredients together for your breakfast smoothie.

8:30 AM – You can start to increase your exercise intensity today if you want if your body feels like it. Remember to always listen to your body during a detox. As long as you don't feel poorly, you can try walking farther or doing a light jog today rather than just doing a simple walk or doing some yoga.

9:00 AM – Take some time to relax and start writing in your detox journal. Now would be a good time to look back over your journey and see how things have been going. You shouldn't be having any side effects and might be feeling pretty good about yourself. Put all these feelings and emotions into your journal. Check on the amount of water you have drunk today and grab a glass if you need to.

9:30 AM – Fix your breakfast burrito and take at least a full 30 minutes to sit an enjoy it. Remember to always pay attention to your food. When you are fully focused on your food, it can help you feel fuller since every part of your body knows that you are eating. Remember to eat slowly as this can help you feel fuller, too. When we eat fast, it can cause us to gain weight because we aren't letting our stomachs have enough time to tell our brains that we are full. You might even think you need more to eat when you really don't.

10:00 AM – If you are taking any supplements, this is the time to take them since you have something on your stomach. Again, check in to make sure you are drinking enough water to reach your goal for a gallon a day.

11:00 AM - Time for your first snack. Since this is almost your last day of the detox, your body might not need this snack. Remember to listen to your body. If you feel like you need this snack, by all means eat it. You might not want it now but might feel a bit hungry later on. That is fine. Just eat when your body tells you it needs it. Continue drinking your water for the day.

11: 15 AM – 12:15 PM – During this time you can do whatever you want. Since this is almost your last day, you can find something fun to do. Do something for yourself. Go to your favorite park, go visit a friend, or just relax with your favorite book. Take some water with you to make sure you are getting all you need.

12:30 PM – It's lunch time. Start making your Portobello mushroom and fennel salad. You can enjoy your meal with a cup of ginger tea if you would like to.

1:30 PM – How is your water intake going? If you are feeling tired of water, you can always choose to have an approved herbal tea if you would like to.

2:00 PM – 3:00 PM – Again check your water level and make sure you are drinking plenty of water. If you have some time, you can write in your detox journal about the progress you have made on this journey.

3:30 PM – Time for your second snack. Again, if you don't feel like you need it, then feel free to skip your snack. Continue drinking your water.

4:00 PM – 5:00 PM – Try for a glass of herbal tea to help get your water intake in. The more you drink during the day, the less you will be faced with at the close of the day.

5:30 PM – Time to fix your dinner. Enjoy your veggie pizza and another big glass of water. Your gallon of water for the day should almost be finished.

6:30 PM – 8:30 PM – If you start to feel hungry at any point during the evening, feel free to snack on some of your approved fruits and veggies.

9:00 PM – Bed – Do whatever you want to help you relax for bed. You can have another glass of warm lime water or some herbal tea. Read a book and do some meditation. The important thing is to make sure that you help your body to relax so that it can easily slip off to sleep for the day. Getting a good night's rest will make the next day a lot easier. You can also write in your journal one more time before you go off to sleep.

Congratulations, you've just finished another day with only one more to go. You can sleep well knowing you are almost at the end of your journey to make your body happier and healthier. Your body is thanking you for what you have done for it. The last day will likely be a breeze. Reading back through your journal might be a fun thing to do. If you ever want to do this detox again, you can reuse the journal and compare your different detoxes to see how they go.

Chapter 11: Detox Day Seven

Congratulations! You've made it to the last day of your detox. You should be feeling pretty good about yourself right now. Depending on what brought you to this detox, you might have noticed some weight loss. Your joints might not be hurting. Your stomach may be feeling better. You probably have more energy than you've had in a long time. You've shouldn't be feeling any more side effects as your body should have adapted by now. You will find the recipes for today below. Just continue to do what you've been doing and you will feel like you have a brand new body.

Remember to start your day with a glass of warm lime water. To help get rid of all those toxins.

Breakfast: Green Smoothie

What You Will Need:

Ice cubes, 3

Tahini butter, 1 tbsp

Hemp seeds, 1 tbsp

Kale, 2 handfuls

Burro banana, 1

Coconut milk, 1 c

What You Will Do:

Begin by peeling and chopping up the banana. Place the banana into a freezer safe bag and place in the freezer until frozen. This will take about four hours. Wash the kale. Remove the stem and give it a rough chop. Once the banana is frozen put it into the blender along with all of the other ingredients. Turn the blender on and let it run until everything is creamy and smooth. Enjoy.

Snack 1: Zucchini Chips

What You Will Need:

Sea salt

Grapeseed oil

Zucchini, 6

What You Will Do:

Start by washing the zucchini. Slice the zucchini into thin strips with either a mandolin or sharp knife. Be careful not to cut yourself if using a mandolin. Be sure to use the vegetable guard. Put the zucchini slices into a bowl. Add in some oil and salt and toss them altogether.

Spread the zucchini over a baking sheet. Make sure that you have your oven at 350. Bake your zucchini chips for 15 minutes. Enjoy.

Lunch: Raw Layered Taco Salad

What You Will Need:

Meat:

Cayenne, to taste

Sea salt, to taste

Oregano, 1 tsp

Onion powder, 1 tsp

Walnuts, .5 c

Macadamia nut cream:

Juice of one key lime

Sea salt, .25 tsp

Water, .75 c

Macadamia nuts, 1 c

Guacamole:

Sea salt, to taste

Juice of one key lime

Onion powder, .5 tsp

Chopped tomato, 1 small

Chopped red onion, .25 c

Avocado, 1

Salsa:

Chopped tomato, 1

Chopped onion, 1

Habanero, 1

Sea salt, .5 tsp

Basil, 1 tsp

Oregano, 1 tsp

Other ingredients:

Dandelion greens

Crackers made from a Dr. Sebi approved grain

What You Will Do:

You need to get the walnuts and macadamia nuts soaking in some water. You will just need to put the walnuts into one bowl and put the macadamia nuts in another. Cover each with water and let them soak for four hours.

For Meat:

After the walnuts have soaked, drain well. Put these into a food processor along with the other ingredients. Pulse a few times until it resembles "meat." Spoon out of food processor and set to the side.

For Cream Sauce:

Drain and rinse the macadamia nuts. Put these into a food processor and pulse a few times until they begin to break down. While the processor is running, pour in the lime juice and about .5 cups water. You can add in more water if the mixture is too thick. Sprinkle in the salt. This sauce needs to be very smooth. It shouldn't be grainy at all. When it is to your desired consistency, pour into a bowl and set to the side.

For Guacamole:

Slice the avocado lengthwise and twist to separate. Carefully remove the seed and scoop out the flesh. Place into a bowl and using a fork, mash into chunks. Add in tomato, onion, onion powder, lime juice, and salt. Stir everything together. Set to the side.

For Salsa:

Wash and chop the tomato and onion. Carefully remove the seeds from the habanero and dice finely. You can either do this by hand or put into a food processor. If doing in a food processor, you will just need to seed the habanero, roughly chop the onion and chunk up the tomato. Add the rest of the ingredients in now and pulse a few times to combine. You can keep this as chunky as you want. If you are doing by hand, chop the onion and tomato and put into a bowl. Add the rest of the ingredients and stir well to combine.

**Make sure to wash your hand thoroughly after touching the habanero. Don't touch your face after handling this pepper. You will regret it.

To Make the Salad:

Place the washed dandelion greens into the bottom of a bowl. Add in .25 cups of the guacamole. Place it in the center of the greens. Add in two tablespoons of the salsa and half of the meat. Pour the cream sauce into a plastic baggie, cut off one corner, and pipe on top of meat. You can garnish this with any leftover onion and tomato. Enjoy with your favorite Dr. Sebi approved crackers.

Snack 2: Veggies and Walnut Hummus

What You Will Need:

Tahini, .25 c

Water, 1 tbsp

Onion powder, 1 tsp

Sea salt, 1.5 tsp

Dry walnuts, 1.25 c

Juice of one key lime

Cayenne, .25 tsp

Olive oil, 3 tbsp

Chopped onion, 2 small

Basil, 1 tsp

Chopped zucchini, 2 c

Sliced bell pepper

Sliced cucumber

What You Will Do:

You will need to put the walnuts into a bowl of warm water and let them sit for two hours. Drain well.

Put the lime juice, olive oil, onion, and zucchini into a blender and turn on blender. Let it go until things begin to incorporate. Turn off blender. Add the walnuts to the blender and turn back on until everything is smooth. Turn off blender. Add in the basil, cayenne, salt, onion powder, and water. Keep blending. Turn off blender and add in the tahini. Give it one last blend to make sure everything is incorporated well.

Pour into a bowl and enjoy will veggies.

Dinner: Lime-Chili Stir Fry

What You Will Need:

Cooked wild rice, 1 c

Cayenne pepper, 1

Achiote seeds, 1 tsp

Juice of one key lime

Ginger root, 1 inch

Kale

Zucchini

Onion

Chayote

Bell pepper

Okra

Mushrooms

What You Will Do

Wash and finely chop the cayenne pepper. Put this into a mortar and pestle along with the achiote seeds. Begin grinding these together. Peel the ginger root by scraping it with a spoon. Finely chop it and add it to the mortar and pestle. Add in lime juice as needed to make it into a sauce. Set this aside to let the flavors blend together.

Let's get the vegetables prepped. Wash and peel the chayote. Slice into quarters and remove seed from center of each. Thinly slice the chayote and set to the side. Wash the zucchini. Cut the zucchini in half and then slice each half into quarters. Slice these as small as you would like. Peel the onion, cut into quarters and slice as small as you want. Wash the kale and remove the stem. Chop into bite size pieces. Wash the okra. Remove the tops and slice thinly. Wipe the mushrooms with a damp paper towel and slice thinly. Wash the bell pepper, take the top off and remove ribs and seeds. Slice thinly.

Place all of the prepped vegetables into a steamer and steam for a few minutes. They need to still be a bit crunchy.

Place the rice into a bowl and put all your cooked veggies on top. Pour over the sauce we made earlier.

You will notice that I didn't give you any quantities for the vegetables. This is because only you know how much you can eat. This recipe is very versatile and you can use as many of the above vegetables as you would like. You can even cook more rice to make it a family meal if you want to.

Step-By-Step Guide

A typical day could go like this.

8:00 AM – This is your last day so you probably know how your day is going to go. You will begin by having your glass of warm lime water. As you are sipping your water, get the ingredients together for your breakfast smoothie.

8:30 AM – You can increase your exercise intensity today if you would want if your body feels like it. Remember to always listen to your body during a detox. As long as you don't feel poorly, you can try jogging today rather than just walking or doing some yoga.

9:00 AM – Take some time to relax and start writing in your detox journal. Now would be a good time to look back over your journey and see how you did. You shouldn't be having any side effects for a while now and might be feeling pretty good about yourself. Put all these feelings and emotions into your journal. Check on the amount of water you have drunk today and grab a glass if you need to.

9:30 AM – Fix your breakfast smoothie and take at least a full 30 minutes to sit an enjoy it. Remember to always pay attention to your food. When you are fully focused on your food, it can help you feel fuller since every part of your body know that you are eating. Remember to eat slowly can help with this too. When we eat fast, it can cause us to gain weight because we aren't letting our stomachs have enough time to tell our brains that we are full. You might even think you need more to eat when you really don't.

10:00 AM – If you are taking any supplements, this is the time to take them since you have something on your stomach. Again, check in to make sure you are drinking enough water to reach your goal for a gallon a day.

11:00 AM - Time for your first snack. Since this is your last day of the detox, your body might not need this snack. Remember to listen to your body. If you feel like you need this snack, by all means eat it. You might not want it now but might feel a bit hungry later on. That is fine. Just eat when your body tells you it needs it. Continue drinking your water for the day.

11: 15 AM – 12:15 PM – During this time you can do whatever you want. Since this is your last day, you can celebrate. Do something fun for yourself. Go to a park, watch your favorite movie, or buy a new outfit. Take some water with you to make sure you are getting all you need.

12:30 PM – It's lunch time. Start making your taco salad. You can enjoy your meal with a cup of Bromide Plus tea if you would like to.

1:30 PM – How is your water intake going? If you are feeling tired of water, you can always choose to have an approved herbal tea if you would like to.

2:00 PM – 3:00 PM – Again check your water level and make sure you are drinking plenty of water. If you have some time, you can write in your detox journal about the progress you have made on this journey.

3:30 PM – Time for your second snack. Again, if you don't feel like you need it, then feel free to skip your snack. Continue drinking your water.

4:00 PM – 5:00 PM – Try for a glass of herbal tea to help get your water intake in. The more you drink during the day, the less you will be faced with at the close of the day.

5:30 PM – Time to fix your dinner. Enjoy your lime chili stir fry and another big glass of water. Your gallon of water for the day should almost be finished.

6:30 PM – 8:30 PM – If you start to feel hungry at any point during the evening, feel free to snack on some of your approved fruits and veggies.

9:00 PM – Bed – Do whatever you want to help you relax for bed. You can have another glass of warm lime water or some herbal tea. Read a book and do some meditation. The important thing is to make sure that you help your body to relax so that it can easily slip off to sleep for the day. Getting a good night's rest will make the next day a lot easier. You can also write in your journal one more time before you go off to sleep.

That's it. You've finished your detox journey. Congratulations, you might have lost some weight. Your achy joints and body might be thanking you for helping them feel better. Your stomach problems might have all disappeared. Your allergies might have even gone away. Take this new body and enjoy the rest of your long, healthy life.

Just because you have finished your detox doesn't mean you get to go back to eating what you did before, at least not right away. If you do, you are going to give your body a shock which will make you feel horrible. You don't want to undo everything you have accomplished, do you?

You can continue to follow Dr. Sebi's diet for as long as you would like or you can slowly reintroduce some of your normal eating habits. Just try to continue to use as many of the foods that Dr. Sebi recommends to keep up all the good work. Since you have cleansed all the caffeine and sugars from your body, you probably don't want to reintroduce your body to those toxins.

Again, congratulations on finishing your detox.

Conclusion

Thank you for making it through to the end of *Dr. Sebi Food List Recipes*, let's hope it was informative and able to provide you with all of the tools you need to achieve your goals whatever they may be.

The next step is to start getting ready for your detox. Remember, during the detox you will be limiting yourself of a lot of things. Your body won't be use to this, so expect a little kickback from it. Things that are worthwhile often aren't easy, so stick with it and power through. You will get through it and you will knock that wall right over. Make sure you follow the information in the first chapter to help get yourself ready for the detox, this will help lessen some of the side effects. Above all, you want to listen to your body. This is meant to help improve your health and not cause you any harm. Stay tuned into your body, always.

Finally, if you found this book useful in any way, a review on Amazon is always appreciated!

Description

If you want to cleanse your body of excess mucus and cleanse your body, then you will want to continue reading.

Dr. Sebi was a naturalist and herbalist that found the secret to unlocking a healthy body. The problem is, the way we live and eat causes an excess of mucus to build up in the bodying. Depending on where it builds up, it will create various diseases. Dr. Sebi figure out that to fix this problem, all we had to do was eat natural foods that alkalize the body. An acidic body is breading grounds for diseases and problems, but an alkaline body makes your body healthy.

Dr. Sebi came up with a diet, which is basically an alkaline diet, which helps to clear out the excess mucus. Some people we will follow his diet for the rest of their lives, especially if they have a chronic disease, and there are some who simply follow his 7-day cleanse from time to time when they feel they need to. It doesn't matter which one you decide to follow since it is up to you and your body, but you may find, after a week on the detox, you may want to continue following Dr. Sebi's diet. This book is here to present to you the detox and food list created by Dr. Sebi. Inside, you will learn:

- The ten commandments of Dr. Sebi

- What you should expect to happen during the detox

- How you should get yourself ready for the detox

- A seven-day-detox plan that includes all of the recipes you will need

- The food list that you make sure you stick to during the diet

… And much more.

If you have been feeling stuck and simply yucky, then your body is screaming at you for this detox. There are a lot of different detoxes out there, and even some premade detox, but this book is here to provide you guidelines that are easy to follow and recipes that won't require anything fancy. Premade detoxes are probably one of the worst things you can do because you don't know what's in it, it's processed, and is likely full of additives that your body doesn't want. With the Dr. Sebi detox, you don't have to worry about that.

This is also a great way to move into following the Dr. Sebi diet, if you are interested in following it long term. Dr. Sebi allows you to take your own health and wellness into your own hands. If you are serious about getting healthy, or at the very least, cleansing toxins and mucus from your body, then the Dr. Sebi detox is for you. Don't want any longer. Scroll up now and click "Buy Now."

Extra content: Explore the collection of books about Dr. Sebi

I wrote this collection in order to reach as many people as possible the knowledge of Dr. Sebi. Do a lot of studies and extract all the information that can lead a person to experience a real change in their life, in a simple way. Here is a preview of what you will find in the rest of the books and you will be able to empirically experience the benefits of following his teachings in   a   complete   way.

Dr. Sebi Treatment and Cures Book:

Dr. Sebi Cure for STDs, Herpes, HIV, Diabetes, Lupus, Hair Loss, Kidney, and Other Diseases

Table of Contents

Introduction

"A healthy body is worth more than any dollar amount. You don't want to be the wealthiest person on a hospital bed." – Dr. Sebi

Congratulations on taking the first steps to improve your health by choosing Dr. Sebi Treatment and Cures Book. In this book, you will learn all of the healing secrets of Dr. Sebi and how they can help you to improve your health.

Throughout this book, we will discuss the various treatment methods laid out by Dr. Sebi to help you recover from STDs, diabetes, hair loss, lupus, and kidney disease. But before we jump into that information, let's take a look at who Dr. Sebi is.

"Healing has to be consistent with life itself. If it isn't, then it is not healing. The components have to be from life." – Dr. Sebi

Dr. Sebi was born as Alfredo Darrington Bowman on November 26, 1933, in Illanga, Honduras. His grandmother taught him about herbal healing. He was self-educated. Dr. Sebi is considered a naturalist, biochemist, herbalist, and pathologist. Over his years, he studied herbs all over North, Central, and South America, Caribbean, and Africa. He developed and unique methodology and approach to healing humans with herbs that are rooted in more than 30 years of experience.

When he moved to the US, he wasn't happy with the modern medical practices that they used to treat things like impotency, diabetes, and asthma. He had been diagnosed with obesity, impotence, diabetes, and asthma, and had undergone many modern medical treatments that did not help him. That's what led him to an herbalist in Mexico, and shortly thereafter, he started his herbal healing practice in New York.

He eventually started a second practice, which he called the USHA Research Institute, in La Ceiba, Honduras. He worked with many well-known celebrities, including Michael Jackson, Eddie Murphy, John Travolta, Steven Seagal, and Lisa Lopes.

Dr. Sebi dedicated more than 30 years of his life to come up with a methodology that he was only able to come up with through years of empirical knowledge. Inspired by all of his own healing knowledge and experience he had learned, he started to share the compounds with other people. This is how he gave birth to Dr. Sebi's Cell Food.

Dr. Sebi passed away on August 9, 2016, from pneumonia.

"Growth is painful, change is painful, but nothing is as painful as staying the same." – Dr. Sebi

Chapter 1:The Dr. Sebi Treatment

The research of Western medicine has stated that diseases are caused by a person being infected by bacteria, viruses, or germs. To help a person overcome this "infestation," doctors provide them with inorganic chemicals. Dr. Sebi's research found the flaws in this premise through simple deductive reasoning. Western medicine has consistently used these same methods, and they have always provided people with the same ineffective results.

Instead, if we look at the African approach to diseases, it opposes Western medicine. The African Bio-mineral Balance rejects the bacteria, virus, and germ theory. Dr. Sebi's research found that diseases are able to grow when the mucous membrane is compromised. For example, if your bronchial tubes have too much mucus, the person is diagnosed with bronchitis. If the mucus is in the lungs, then they have pneumonia. When it moves to the pancreatic duct, they have diabetes. All of the compounds in the African Bio-mineral Balance are made up of natural plants, which make it alkaline.

This is very important in reversing these pathologies because diseases are only able to live in acidic environments. It doesn't make sense to use inorganic compounds to treat diseases because they are acidic. The consistent use of natural remedies will detoxify and cleanse a diseased body and will bring it back to its alkaline state.

Dr. Sebi's nutrition system takes things a step further. Besides getting rid of years of toxin build-up, the African Bio-mineral Balance will replace all of the depleted minerals and will rejuvenate any cell tissue that has been damaged by acid. The main organs that it helps are the colon, kidneys, lymph glands, gall bladder, liver, and skin. When the toxins are released from one of these organs, they will move through the body and manifest in disease. Eventually, the body will start to attack the weakest organ because it is unable to get rid of the toxin. The colon is probably one of the most important organs and needs to be cleansed before diseases are able to be reversed. But, if you only cleanse the colon, all of the other organs will still be toxic, which leaves the body diseased.

Through Dr. Sebi's intra-cellular detoxifying cleanse, every cell within the body will be purified. The body is then able to rejuvenate and rebuild itself.

Dr. Sebi's Diet

The Dr. Sebi diet is a plant-based alkaline diet. It helps to rejuvenate the cells in your body by getting rid of the toxic waste. The bulk of the diet is made up of a shortlist of foods along with supplements.

Dr. Sebi's diet is also able to help conditions like lupus, AIDS, kidney disease, and other diseases. The treatments for these diseases require you to eat only certain grains, fruits, and veggies, and strictly abstaining from animal products.

This is a very low protein diet, and that's what makes Dr. Sebi's supplements so important. You cannot have soy or animal products, lentils, or beans. You have several different options when it comes to Dr. Sebi's supplement choices, and you can even purchase and "all-inclusive" package that has 20 different products and can help to restore your body's health.

If you don't want to do the "all-inclusive" package, you can pick supplements according to the health problems you are suffering from. For example, Bio Ferro can help to increase overall wellbeing, help digestive issues, promote weight loss, boost immunity, cleanse the blood, and treat liver problems.

Weight Loss

While Dr. Sebi's diet isn't meant to be a weight loss diet, it can help you to lose weight. Since you will be cutting out all of the processed foods that most Western diets are made of, as well as fats, sugar, salt, and calories, you will likely lose weight.

Dr. Sebi's diet is a plant-based, vegan diet, and people who follow a plant-based diet often have a lower rate of heart disease and obesity. Plus, most of the foods you are allowed to eat are low in calories, except for oils, avocados, seeds, and nut, so even if you were to eat a lot of these foods, it is very unlikely that you are going to gain weight.

Benefits

Since you will be consuming a large number of fruits and veggies, it provides your body with many health benefits. Diets that are rich in fruits and veggies have been connected to less oxidative stress and reduced inflammation and can help to protect you from many different diseases.

Dr. Sebi's diet will also have you eating healthy fats and fiber-rich whole grains. All of these foods are connected to a lower risk of heart disease. Plus, you will be limiting those horrible processed foods, which is connected to better overall diet quality.

The biggest issue, though, that people have with Dr. Sebi's diet is that it is very restrictive and cuts out entire food groups that most people are used to eating. Plus, it can get very restrictive on the types of fruit and vegetables you are allowed to eat. Some people may struggle with this, but with some guidance and planning, you can make the switch.

Dr. Sebi Recipe Book:

101 Tasty and Easy-Made Cell Foods for Detox, Cleanse, and Revitalizing Your Body and Soule Using the Dr. Sebi Food List and Products

Table of Contents

Avocado Basil Pasta Salad

Veggie Pizza

Lasagna

Kale and Brazil Nut Pesto with Butternut Squash

Zoodles in Avocado Sauce

Fried Rice

Rice and Spinach Balls

Flatbread

Chickpea "Tuna" Salad

Enoki Mushroom Pasta

Pasta with Walnut Pesto

Vegetable Alfredo

Mushroom Stroganoff

Walnut Kale Pasta

Tomato Pasta

Spicy Sesame Ginger Noodle Bowl

Zucchini Tomato Pasta

Creamy Mushroom Pasta

Creamy Kamut Pasta

Chicken and Waffles

Quiche

Macaroni and Cheese

Ravioli

Wraps and Sandwiches

Nori-Burritos

Grilled Zucchini and Hummus Wrap

Portobello Burgers

Veggie Fajitas

Spelt Bread

Chickpea Burger

Mushroom Cheese Steak

Squash Falafels

Home Fries

Chicken Tenders

Hot Dogs

Spring Rolls

Cereals

Hummus

Crunchy Hummus

Vegetable Quinoa

Kamut Cereal

Kamut Puff Cereal

Teff Porridge

Quinoa Cereal

Green Detox

Iron Power

Sweet Sunrise

Coconut Lime

Super Shake

Alkaline Smoothie

Apple Banana

Mango Strawberry

Strawberry Banana Quinoa

Glowing Green Smoothie

Alkaline Boosting Smoothie

Aloha Breakfast Smoothie

Green Detox Smoothie

Avocado Detox

Pumpkin Spice Smoothie

Summer Berry

Liquid Fat-Burning Smoothie

Hearty Power Smoothie

Berry Good Kale Smoothie

Tahini Butter Crunch Smoothie

Raspberry Lime Smoothie

"Cinnamon" Bun Smoothie

Summer Citrus Smoothie

Lean, Green Protein Smoothie

Spring Ahead Smoothie

Blueberry Morning Blast

Blackberry Smoothie

Winter Green Smoothie

Coco Loco Smoothie

Glorious Breakfast Smoothie

Berry Peach Smoothie

Apple Pie

Veggie-Ful

Energizing

Tropical Breeze

Super Hydrating

Sea Moss Green

Mango Banana

Kale Berry Delight

Banana Coconut

Apple Juice Mix

Banana Flax

Fresh Greens

Banana Berry Kale

Mucus Cleanse Tea

ImmuniTea

Ginger Turmeric Tea

Tranquil Tea

Energizing Lemon Tea

Pregnan-Tea

Respiratory Support Tea

Thyme and Lemon Tea

Sore Throat Tea

Autumn Tonic Tea

Adrenal and Stress Health

Lavender Tea

Rosy Black Tea

Tranquil Tea

Soothing Lemon Tea

Morning Refresher

Berry Lime Tea

Zestea

Feminine Balance Tea

Pregnancy-Safe Headache Tea

Teething Tea

Ginger Shot

Introduction

I would like to thank you for choosing *Dr. Sebi Recipe Book*. This book will provide you with 101 delicious recipes that you can enjoy as you follow Dr. Sebi's diet.

For those of you who do not know, Dr. Sebi was a naturalist, biochemist, herbalist, and pathologist. During his life, he studied herbs throughout the Caribbean, Africa, and all of America. Through his studies, he came up with his own methodology and approach to healing the body with herbs.

He was born on November 26, 1933, as Alfredo Bowman in Ilanga Village in Honduras. He was completely self-educated and learned a lot from his grandmother. During his childhood, he would play in the forest and by the river and learned a lot about nature.

After he made his move to the United States, he was diagnosed with obesity, impotency, diabetes, and asthma, but modern medicine couldn't help him. This led him to travel to Mexico to see an herbalist. He found great success with this route, and he started to create natural methods of healing the cells in the body. He dedicated more than 30 years of his life coming up with his own methodology. This is how he gave birth to Dr. Sebi's Cell Food.

His teachings have disputed germ theory. Dr. Sebi did not believe that our ailments were caused by germs, bacteria, viruses, and so on. He believed that the root of all of our problems was an excess of mucus in the system. Many of his teachings were Afrocentric and focused on the unique genetic characteristics of Africans.

Dr. Sebi had a practice in New York and then opened USHA Research Institute in Usha Village in Honduras. Throughout his years, he has worked with lots of celebrities. Wendy Williams once took her son, Kevin Jr., to Usha Village to help him after he used synthetic marijuana.

TLCs Lisa Lopes also visited Usha Village during her short time. This was also where she had been when she was in her unfortunate accident. He also helped treat Michael Jackson, Nipsey Hussle, John Travolta, Steven Seagal, and Eddie Murphy.

In 1988, Dr. Sebi was faced with a Supreme Court trial for false advertisement and practicing without a license. This happened after he had placed ads in several newspapers. The judge asked Dr. Sebi to produce one person for each disease. He said that he could cure. When the trial started, Dr. Sebi brought in 77 people. The juror ended up ruling in his favor and found him not guilty. After this, he moved his practice to LA.

He continued to thrive even after the lawsuit. Unfortunately, he was faced with another lawsuit. He was arrested on May 28, 2016, in Honduras for money laundering. He was never able to defend himself in this matter because he died of complications with pneumonia at the age of 82 while in police custody.

Despite these setbacks, Dr. Sebi still lives on in the hearts of those he has helped and continues to help.

Chapter 1: Eating Naturally with Dr. Sebi's Teachings

The Dr. Sebi diet is often referred to as the African biomineral balance. This was how he would cure people of a variety of diseases. It is basically a vegan diet that is made up of foods that he called "electric" or alkaline foods. It is suggested that, while following this diet, you also take his healing supplements.

You cannot eat any meat or animal products while on this diet, as well as foods that contain a lot of starch. The reason for this is that you are only supposed to eat alkaline-forming foods, and those foods form acids.

Meat products cause uric acid production, dairy produces cause lactic acid, and starch causes carbonic acid. All of these acids will build-up, which causes a buildup of mucus. The mucus robs our cells of oxygen. However, if you eat electric foods, they feed the body. The human body is electrical, so it needs electric food to function.

This diet is made up of grains, teas, nuts, veggies, and fruits. Among the foods you can eat are wild rice, amaranth, quinoa, mushrooms, watercress, kale, dates, figs, mangos, avocados, and much more. These foods will help to nourish your body and won't end up causing an accumulation of mucus.

If you plan on really starting this diet, you must make sure that you really want it. The first thing you will need to do is to make some changes to how you eat. You will probably find that this is going to require you to be your best emotional state and the right state of mind.

Eating is a big part of our life, and the types of things we consume form strong habits that can end up lasting our entire life. It can be very hard to break these habits and deal with the influence of family and friends. That means, before you jump right into this diet, you should take some time thinking about changing how you eat. You don't want to promise yourself this and then end up not being able to follow through just because you weren't prepared.

Instead, you should begin slowly. You can even talk to your family and friends. The reaction you can get from people when you talk to them about Dr. Sebi's diet will vary. Some will want to learn more, while others will write it off as bunk.

That being said, you shouldn't tire yourself by trying to convince everybody else before you make sure that it is right for you. Your vitality, health improvements, and cleaner outlook will show your family way more than just your words.

Once you do start making the transition, the first thing you need to do is to start reading food ingredient labels on everything. This will help you to stay conscious about what you are drinking and eating. When you are first starting out, before you live completely by the nutritional guide, this awareness is going to provide you with the incentive to change things as you continue on. Later on, if you do end up straying from the diet, you will still be able to remain conscious about what you are eating.

If you have long been a meat-eater, that may be the hardest thing to transition from. The best thing you can do is to start making the transition from meats by switching to eating only fish. Then you can slowly start eating less and less fish each week.

It is also important that you start making your own snacks. This will ensure if you do get the urge to snack, that you will have good snacks to eat. Approved nuts and raisins are a good choice.

Then you need to make sure that you are eating all of the correct foods. That means you need to learn what foods are and aren't on the nutritional guide. You must stick to only those foods. At first, this will feel tough, and that is expected. In fact, it is very hard to do in our society when only the bad foods are pushed at us. This is the reason why I stressed that you must be emotionally ready.

You also need to make sure you are drinking plenty of water. While we have all known for a while now that water is a very important part of our health, most of us are still not drink enough. Plus, there are a lot of Dr. Sebi products that you will be taking, like the Bromide Plus Powder, contain herbs that act as diuretics. That means you have to take extra care to make sure you don't allow yourself to get dehydrated.

Dr. Sebi suggests that you drink a gallon of spring water every day. Springwater has a natural alkaline pH, whereas tap water can be high in chloride and many other contaminants.

You will also need to learn how to cook your own meals if you don't cook already. You aren't going to find too many prepackaged foods that fit into the Dr. Sebi diet. Once you do get the hang of cooking, you will find that you can change your favorite dishes into Dr. Sebi-approved dishes.